365 Days of Self-Care for 2026

Simple Daily Practices for Peace, Balance, and Personal Renewal

Stephen D. Arkwillow

Copyright

Disclaimer

This book is intended for inspirational and educational purposes only. It is not a substitute for professional medical, psychological, legal, or therapeutic advice, diagnosis, or treatment. The reflections and practices offered are designed to support personal awareness, self-care, and emotional well-being, but they are not intended to address or resolve clinical conditions.

Readers are encouraged to use their own judgment and to consult qualified professionals regarding any physical, mental, or emotional health concerns. The author and publisher assume no responsibility for any outcomes resulting from the use or application of the information contained in this book.

Every individual's experience is unique. What feels supportive or meaningful for one person may not feel the same for another. Readers are invited to engage with the content at their own pace, adapting or skipping any practice that does not feel appropriate for them.

By reading this book, you acknowledge that you are responsible for your own well-being and choices, and you agree to use the material in a way that respects your personal needs and circumstances.

Table of Contents

Introduction

This book is not about becoming someone new. It is about caring for who you already are.

Self-care is often presented as something to master, schedule, or optimize. In reality, it is quieter than that. It lives in the small choices you make when no one is watching, in how you speak to yourself when you are tired, and in whether you allow yourself to pause without justification. This book was created as a companion for those moments.

You do not need to be overwhelmed, broken, or struggling to begin. You only need a willingness to meet yourself where you are. Each day in this book offers a short reflection meant to be read slowly, held briefly, and then lived in your own way. Nothing here is meant to be forced or completed perfectly. Some days you may read only a few lines. Other days you may return to a page more than once. Both are enough.

The structure of this book follows the natural rhythm of a year. Some months focus on grounding and clarity, others on growth, rest, connection, or renewal. This progression is intentional, but it is not rigid. Life rarely unfolds in straight lines, and self-care does not either. You are welcome to move through the book at your own pace, revisit pages that resonate, or skip days that do not feel relevant in the moment.

These daily reflections are not instructions or solutions. They are gentle invitations. Each one is designed to fit into five to ten minutes of your day, offering space to breathe, reflect, and respond with care. There is no requirement to journal, analyze, or achieve. Simply noticing and allowing is enough.

As you move through the year, you may begin to notice subtle shifts. A softer inner voice. A clearer sense of what you need. A greater ability to rest without guilt or to act without rushing. These changes are not dramatic, and they are not meant to be. Self-care works best when it is quiet, consistent, and kind.

This book is yours. Use it in the way that feels most supportive to you. Let it sit on your bedside table, your desk, or anywhere you return to regularly.

Open it on difficult days and ordinary ones alike. There is no right way to move through these pages, only an honest one.

May this book remind you, again and again, that caring for yourself is not selfish or indulgent. It is necessary. It is allowed. And it can begin today, exactly as you are.

JANUARY

Reset & Intention

Reset, readjust, restart, refocus as many times as you need to.
—Unknown

January arrives quietly. It does not demand that you become someone new or leave parts of yourself behind. Instead, it offers you space—space to pause, to notice, and to begin again without judgment.

This month is about resetting your relationship with yourself. Not through pressure or strict resolutions, but through honest attention. Resetting means allowing yourself to arrive fully in the present moment, exactly as you are, before deciding where to go next. Intention, here, is not about control. It is about care.

Throughout January, you are invited to slow down enough to hear yourself again. To recognize your needs without immediately dismissing them. To take small, steady steps that rebuild trust between your body, your mind, and your inner life.

There is no race to win this month. There is only the practice of beginning—gently, truthfully, and with compassion.

JANUARY 1

Begin Where You Are

There is often a quiet pressure at the start of a new year to move forward quickly—to plan, to fix, to improve. Today asks you to resist that pull and do something far more grounding: begin exactly where you are.

Before looking ahead, take a moment to notice your present state. How does your body feel right now? Where are you holding tension, if any? What emotions are closest to the surface as this year begins? There is no need to analyze or label them. Simply noticing is enough.

Beginning where you are does not mean settling or giving up. It means rooting yourself in honesty. When you acknowledge your current reality without judgment, you create a stable place from which real change can grow. Growth that is forced tends to fracture. Growth that is grounded tends to last.

Spend five quiet minutes today sitting or standing still. Place your feet firmly on the floor. Let your breath move naturally. If your thoughts wander, gently bring them back to the sensation of being here, now. Nothing needs to be solved in this moment.

As you move through the rest of the day, return to this reminder whenever you feel behind or uncertain:

I am allowed to begin exactly where I am.

JANUARY 2

Breathe Before You Rush

Rushing often begins before anything has actually gone wrong. It starts as a subtle tightening in the body, a quickening of thoughts, a sense that you are already behind. Today invites you to interrupt that pattern in the simplest way possible—by returning to your breath.

Before you move into the demands of the day, pause for a moment. Notice where you are breathing. Is it shallow or deep? Fast or slow? Without trying to fix it, allow one full breath to move gently in and out. Let your shoulders drop. Let your jaw soften. This is not about doing breathing "correctly." It is about remembering that you have a choice.

Throughout the day, especially when you feel pressure rising, come back to this pause. Even one conscious breath creates space. It slows the moment just enough for you to respond with clarity instead of momentum. You do not need to match the pace of the world around you. You are allowed to move at a rhythm that feels sustainable.

Take five minutes today to practice this intentionally. Sit or stand comfortably and take several slow, natural breaths, noticing the quiet steadiness beneath the movement. Let your breath remind you that you are here, supported, and not required to rush through your life.

As you carry this into the rest of the day, return to this grounding thought whenever you feel hurried:
I breathe first, and then I move.

JANUARY 3

Choose One Gentle Intention

Intentions are often confused with expectations. Today invites you to release that confusion and approach intention as something softer—something that guides rather than demands. A gentle intention does not push you forward. It walks beside you.

Take a moment this morning to ask yourself how you want to *feel* today, not what you want to accomplish. Calm, steady, patient, open, present—let the word that feels most supportive rise naturally. There is no need to force an answer. Trust what comes easily.

Once you have chosen your intention, hold it lightly. Let it be something you return to when the day feels scattered or heavy. If you forget it, that is not a failure. Simply remembering again is part of the practice.

Spend a few minutes writing your intention down or repeating it quietly to yourself. Notice how it settles in your body. Let it shape your day gently, without pressure.

As you move forward today, remind yourself:
My intention supports me, it does not control me.

JANUARY 4

Create a Calm Morning Moment

The way you enter your day sets a tone that often lingers longer than you realize. Today is not about creating a perfect morning routine, but about carving out one calm moment that belongs only to you.

This moment does not need to be long. It may be sitting quietly before checking your phone, taking a few slow breaths while the day wakes up, or standing near a window and noticing the light. What matters is presence, not productivity.

Allow this moment to be free of goals. You are not preparing yourself to perform. You are simply allowing yourself to arrive. When mornings begin with even a small sense of calm, the rest of the day often feels more manageable.

Give yourself five minutes today to begin gently. Let that calm accompany you as you move into what comes next.

Carry this reminder with you:

I am allowed to begin my day with ease.

JANUARY 5

Clear One Small Space

Clutter often takes up more mental space than we realize. Today invites you to clear just one small area—not as a task to complete, but as an act of care.

Choose something manageable: a drawer, a bag, a surface. Move slowly as you sort. Notice what feels necessary and what feels ready to be released. There is no right outcome. The intention is not perfection, but relief.

As you create physical space, pay attention to how your body responds. Many people notice a quiet sense of lightness or clarity. Let that feeling register.

This small act is a reminder that you have the ability to create ease, one step at a time.

As you finish, reflect on this thought:
I make room for what supports me.

JANUARY 6

Listen to Your Inner Pace

Your body carries its own wisdom about speed. Today invites you to listen to it instead of overriding it.

Notice when you feel rushed and when you feel settled. Notice how your energy rises and falls throughout the day. None of this needs correction. Awareness is the goal.

If you are able, adjust your pace slightly—walking a bit slower, pausing between tasks, allowing transitions instead of rushing through them. These small shifts often reduce tension more than we expect.

Give yourself permission to move at a pace that feels sustainable, not impressive.

Return to this truth today:
 My natural pace deserves respect.

JANUARY 7

Release Pressure to Perfect

Perfection often disguises itself as responsibility, but it usually carries tension beneath it. Today invites you to notice where you may be holding yourself to standards that leave little room to breathe.

Ask yourself where "good enough" might actually be enough. Where could you soften without things falling apart? Often, releasing perfection does not lead to failure—it leads to relief.

Spend a few moments today consciously allowing something to be incomplete or imperfect. Notice how it feels in your body when you let go of tightening control.

Perfection is not required for worth or care.

Hold this thought gently:
I release the need to be perfect.

JANUARY 8

Nourish Yourself First

It is easy to move through the day giving your energy outward before checking in with yourself. Today invites you to pause and notice whether you are tending to your own needs or quietly pushing past them. Nourishment is not something to postpone until everything else is finished.

Take a moment to notice what your body is asking for right now. You may feel thirsty, tired, tense, or simply in need of quiet. These signals are not interruptions; they are information meant to guide you back to balance.

Choose one small way to nourish yourself before continuing with the day. It might be drinking water slowly, taking a few steady breaths, or allowing yourself a brief pause without distraction. Let the act be simple and intentional.

When you nourish yourself first, you support your ability to stay present and steady throughout the day. Care offered early does not take away from others—it strengthens what you can give.

I am worthy of nourishment.

JANUARY 9

Practice Kind Self-Talk

Your inner voice shapes how you experience each moment, often more powerfully than outside circumstances. Today invites you to listen to how you speak to yourself, especially when things feel difficult or imperfect. Awareness is the first step toward softness.

Notice moments when your thoughts become critical or impatient. Pause and ask yourself what tone would feel more supportive. Kind self-talk does not excuse mistakes; it creates safety while you learn and adjust.

Practice offering yourself the same understanding you would give someone you care about. Even one gentle response can ease tension and shift how your body holds the moment.

Throughout the day, return to kindness when you notice harshness creeping in. Small shifts in

language create lasting changes over time.
I speak to myself with care.

JANUARY 10

Notice What Brings Ease

Ease often goes unnoticed because it does not demand attention. Today invites you to slow down just enough to recognize moments when your body or mind feels lighter, calmer, or more settled. These moments are worth noticing.

Pay attention to subtle signs of ease—a relaxed breath, a softening in your shoulders, a task that flows without resistance. Let yourself pause with that feeling instead of rushing past it.

Ease is not something you must earn or justify. It is a natural state that becomes more accessible when you stop pushing yourself unnecessarily. Allow yourself to trust what feels supportive.

As you move through the day, let ease guide your choices where possible. It can quietly point you toward balance.

I allow myself to notice what feels easy.

JANUARY 11

Rest Without Earning It

Rest is often treated as something that must be justified, as if you need to prove exhaustion before allowing yourself to pause. Today invites you to question that belief and consider rest as a natural part of caring for yourself, not a reward for productivity.

Notice where you may be pushing past signs of fatigue, telling yourself you will rest later. These small dismissals add up over time, quietly draining your energy and patience. Rest does not need a reason beyond the fact that you are human.

Allow yourself a moment of rest today without explanation or apology. It may be a few quiet minutes, a slower pace, or simply stopping when you notice tension building. Let rest be intentional rather than accidental.

When you allow rest without conditions, your body and mind respond with steadiness instead of strain. I am allowed to rest.

JANUARY 12

Set One Honest Boundary

Boundaries are not walls meant to keep others out; they are guidelines that protect your energy and well-being. Today invites you to notice where you feel stretched too thin or quietly uncomfortable, and to respond with honesty.

Pause and ask yourself what boundary would feel supportive right now. It might be saying no, asking for space, or allowing yourself to stop before exhaustion sets in. Let the boundary be clear but gentle.

Setting a boundary may feel uncomfortable at first, especially if you are used to prioritizing others. With time, boundaries create more ease, not less, by honoring your limits.

Today, remind yourself that boundaries are a form of care, not conflict.

My boundaries support my well-being.

JANUARY 13

Drink Water With Awareness

Today's practice is simple and grounding, yet often overlooked. Drinking water with awareness brings you back into your body and into the present moment, even during a busy day.

As you drink, notice the temperature, the sensation, and the way your body responds. Let this moment be unhurried. There is no need to multitask or rush through it.

This small act of attention is a quiet reminder that your body has needs worth listening to. Awareness turns an ordinary action into an act of care.

As you hydrate today, return to this gentle thought:
 I care for my body with attention.

JANUARY 14

Start Again Without Guilt

There are moments when plans fall apart, intentions slip, or days don't unfold as expected. Today invites you to release the weight of guilt that often follows and to remember that starting again is always available.

Notice where you may be holding onto disappointment or self-blame. Guilt does not help you move forward; compassion does. Starting again does not erase progress—it continues it.

Allow yourself to reset today without explaining or justifying the restart. Each moment offers a fresh beginning, no matter how many times you need it.

Carry this reminder gently through the day:
I am allowed to begin again.

JANUARY 15

Simplify Today's Expectations

Expectations can quietly pile up until they feel heavy and overwhelming. Today invites you to look at what you expect of yourself and to gently simplify where possible.

Ask yourself what truly needs to be done today, and what can be softened or postponed. Let go of unnecessary pressure that does not serve your well-being.

Simplifying expectations is not about doing less out of avoidance. It is about choosing clarity over overwhelm and intention over strain.

As you move through the day, return to this grounding thought:
 I choose simplicity over pressure.

JANUARY 16

Allow Yourself to Move Slowly

Moving slowly can feel uncomfortable in a world that rewards speed and constant motion, yet today invites you to notice how often rushing happens automatically rather than out of true necessity or care.

Slowing down does not mean losing direction or falling behind, but instead gives your body and mind the space they need to stay present rather than continually recovering from urgency.

Choose one part of your day to move more slowly, whether that means walking with awareness, pausing between tasks, or allowing transitions to unfold without pressure or self-criticism.

As you move through the day, let this reminder settle gently within you:
I am allowed to move at a pace that supports me.

JANUARY 17

Name What You Truly Need

Your needs often make themselves known quietly through tension, fatigue, or restlessness, and today invites you to pause long enough to listen without immediately dismissing or judging what you hear.

Naming a need does not mean it must be solved right away, but it does allow you to acknowledge what is true beneath the surface and to meet yourself with honesty rather than avoidance.

Spend a few moments checking in with yourself and gently naming one need, allowing it to exist without pressure, explanation, or comparison to what others may expect.

Carry this truth with you throughout the day:
My needs are valid and worthy of attention.

JANUARY 18

Let Go of Yesterday's Weight

Yesterday can linger in subtle ways, showing up as tension in the body or repeated thoughts that quietly pull your attention backward instead of allowing you to arrive fully today.

Letting go does not require forgetting or minimizing what happened, but it does involve choosing not to carry its emotional weight forward into moments that deserve fresh space.

Take a brief pause today to imagine setting down what no longer needs to follow you, allowing your breath and body to respond to the release.

As you step into the rest of the day, remind yourself:
I allow today to stand on its own.

JANUARY 19

Make Time for Stillness

Stillness can feel unfamiliar when life is full, yet it offers a quiet counterbalance that helps restore clarity, steadiness, and a sense of internal grounding.

Stillness does not require silence or long stretches of time, but instead can be found in a few deliberate breaths or a pause taken before responding or moving on.

Allow yourself one moment of intentional stillness today, letting it be enough without turning it into another task or obligation.

Hold this reminder gently as you continue:
I make room for stillness.

JANUARY 20

Do One Thing Mindfully

Mindfulness does not need to shape your entire day to be meaningful, as even one fully attended moment can anchor you more deeply in the present.

Choose a single activity today and give it your full attention, noticing sensations and movements while allowing distractions to pass without frustration.

This brief act of presence can quietly shift how the rest of your day feels, offering steadiness rather than strain.

Let this thought guide you forward:
This moment is enough.

JANUARY 21

Welcome Support From Others

There is often an unspoken belief that needing support is a sign of weakness, yet today invites you to reconsider that idea and recognize support as a natural part of being human.

Support may already exist around you in quiet ways, through listening, shared presence, or small acts of kindness that do not require explanation or repayment.

Allow yourself to receive support today without minimizing your needs or rushing to prove independence, noticing how your body responds when you are not carrying everything alone.

As you move through the day, let this truth guide you:
I am allowed to be supported.

JANUARY 22

Honor Your Energy Levels

Your energy is not constant, and today invites you to notice its natural rhythm rather than pushing yourself to maintain the same pace regardless of how you feel.

Honoring your energy means listening when your body asks for rest or adjustment, even if your plans or expectations suggest otherwise.

Choose one small way to work with your energy today instead of against it, allowing flexibility where you can and softness where you need it.

Carry this reminder gently with you:
I respect my energy and capacity.

JANUARY 23

Choose Calm Over Urgency

Urgency often creates the illusion that everything must happen immediately, yet today invites you to pause and notice whether calm might serve you better in this moment.

Calm does not mean ignoring responsibility, but it does allow you to respond with clarity rather than reacting from pressure or fear.

Take one intentional pause today before responding or deciding, letting your breath create space between the moment and your action.

As you continue, remember:
I choose calm when it is available.

JANUARY 24

Create a Simple Evening Ritual

The way you end your day quietly shapes how your body and mind settle into rest, and today invites you to create a simple ritual that signals closure and care.

This ritual does not need to be elaborate, but should feel comforting and intentional, offering a gentle transition from doing to being.

Allow yourself to repeat this ritual without rushing, letting it mark the end of effort and the beginning of rest.

As night arrives, hold this thought softly:
I allow my day to end gently.

JANUARY 25

Trust Small Consistent Steps

Change is often imagined as dramatic or immediate, yet today invites you to notice the quiet strength of small actions repeated with care.

Consistency does not require intensity, but rather a willingness to show up in manageable ways that support steadiness over time.

Reflect on one small step you have taken recently and allow yourself to acknowledge its value without minimizing it.

Let this reminder accompany you:
I trust the process of small steps.

JANUARY 26

Speak Gently to Yourself

The tone you use with yourself influences how safe and supported you feel internally, and today invites you to soften that tone wherever possible.

Notice moments when your inner dialogue becomes sharp or impatient, and pause to offer yourself a gentler response instead.

Speaking kindly to yourself does not remove challenges, but it does change how you carry them through the day.

Return to this thought when needed:
I choose gentleness with myself.

JANUARY 27

Pause Before Reacting

Reactions often happen faster than awareness, yet today invites you to introduce a pause that creates choice and clarity.

This pause may be as brief as a single breath, but it can shift how you respond and how your body holds the moment.

Allow yourself to practice this pause today, especially when emotions feel strong or situations feel tense.

Hold this reminder gently:
I pause before I respond.

JANUARY 28

Make Space for Quiet Joy

Joy does not always arrive loudly or dramatically, and today invites you to notice quieter moments of contentment that often pass unnoticed.

These moments may appear as comfort, ease, or simple appreciation, asking only to be acknowledged rather than analyzed.

Allow yourself to linger briefly with quiet joy today, letting it register without questioning whether it is deserved.

Carry this thought with you:
I allow joy to be simple.

JANUARY 29

Reflect on What's Working

Reflection helps bring awareness to progress that can be overlooked when attention stays fixed on what feels unfinished.

Today invites you to notice what is supporting you right now, even if it feels small or ordinary.

Allow yourself to acknowledge what works without dismissing it or rushing past the recognition.

As you continue, remember:
I notice what supports me.

JANUARY 30

Release What No Longer Fits

Some things quietly outgrow their place in your life, and today invites you to notice what may be ready to be released.

Letting go does not require force or finality, but rather a gentle willingness to stop carrying what feels heavy or outdated.

Take a moment to imagine setting something down, trusting that space itself can be supportive.

Hold this reminder today:
 I let go with care.

JANUARY 31

Step Forward With Intention

As January comes to a close, today invites you to pause and notice what this month has offered you rather than rushing toward what comes next.

Stepping forward with intention does not require certainty, only a willingness to move with awareness and care into the days ahead.

Reflect briefly on what you want to carry forward, allowing it to guide you quietly rather than dictate your path.

As you move on, hold this truth gently:
I step forward with intention.

FEBRUARY

Self-Compassion & Care

You yourself, as much as anybody in the entire universe, deserve your love and affection.
—Buddha

February invites a softer kind of attention, one that turns inward with patience rather than judgment, and asks how you might care for yourself in the same way you instinctively care for others.

This month is not about fixing what you believe is wrong with you, but about meeting yourself honestly, especially in moments when you feel tired, imperfect, or unsure.

Self-compassion is not indulgence or avoidance, but a steady willingness to stay present with yourself without withdrawing warmth when things feel difficult.

As you move through these days, allow care to feel simple, human, and deserved, even when old habits tell you otherwise.

FEBRUARY 1

Treat Yourself Like a Friend

You likely offer patience, encouragement, and understanding to the people you care about, yet today invites you to notice whether you extend that same generosity toward yourself.

Treating yourself like a friend means listening without interruption, responding without harshness, and allowing room for mistakes without attaching shame or disappointment.

Throughout the day, notice moments when you speak to yourself sharply, and gently ask how you would respond if someone you loved were in the same situation.

Let this practice guide you today as a quiet standard of care:
I treat myself with the same kindness I offer others.

FEBRUARY 2

Soften Self-Criticism

Self-criticism often arises automatically, shaped by long-held habits rather than present truth, and today invites you to notice its tone without immediately agreeing with it.

Softening self-criticism does not mean ignoring responsibility, but it does mean choosing curiosity and care instead of judgment when things feel difficult.

When you catch a critical thought today, pause briefly and offer a gentler alternative that acknowledges effort rather than focusing only on shortcomings.

Carry this reminder with you as the day unfolds:
I can be honest without being harsh.

FEBRUARY 3

Allow Imperfection Today

There is quiet pressure to appear capable, composed, and consistent, yet today invites you to allow imperfection without apology or explanation.

Imperfection does not mean failure, but evidence that you are participating fully in life rather than trying to control every outcome.

Notice moments when something feels unfinished or messy, and resist the urge to correct it immediately unless it truly needs attention.

Let this truth settle gently within you today:
I am allowed to be imperfect.

FEBRUARY 4

Rest Your Mind Briefly

Your mind carries more than it often reveals, and today invites you to give it a brief rest from constant planning, reviewing, and problem-solving.

Resting your mind does not require silence or long breaks, but can be found in a few moments of focused breathing or gentle awareness.

Allow yourself to step out of mental effort briefly, trusting that clarity often returns more easily after rest than force.

As you move forward, remember:
My mind is allowed to rest.

FEBRUARY 5

Accept Your Feelings Fully

Feelings often come with an impulse to fix, justify, or push them away, yet today invites you to allow them to exist without resistance.

Accepting feelings does not mean acting on them, but it does mean acknowledging their presence without judgment or urgency.

Pause today when emotions arise and allow them space, noticing how acceptance often softens intensity rather than increasing it.

Let this reminder accompany you gently:
My feelings are allowed to exist.

FEBRUARY 6

Choose Warmth Over Judgment

Judgment can arise quickly, especially toward yourself, yet today invites you to choose warmth as your first response whenever possible.

Warmth does not remove accountability, but it creates an internal environment where learning and growth feel safer and more sustainable.

Notice moments when judgment appears, and consciously soften your inner response with understanding instead of critique.

Hold this truth close today:
Warmth supports me better than judgment.

FEBRUARY 7

Forgive Yourself Gently

Forgiveness is often imagined as something dramatic, yet today invites you to practice it gently, in small moments where self-blame quietly lingers.

Forgiving yourself does not erase responsibility, but it does release the ongoing punishment that prevents healing and forward movement.

Take a moment today to acknowledge something you've been holding against yourself, and allow compassion to replace repetition.

Let this thought guide you forward:
I forgive myself with care.

FEBRUARY 8

Practice Loving Inner Talk

The way you speak to yourself throughout the day quietly shapes how safe and supported you feel internally, and today invites you to become more aware of that inner conversation.

Loving inner talk does not mean constant positivity, but rather responding to yourself with patience, reassurance, and respect when things feel uncertain or difficult.

Notice moments when your inner voice becomes demanding or dismissive, and gently offer yourself language that feels more understanding and steady.

As you move through the day, return to this reminder:
I speak to myself with warmth and care.

FEBRUARY 9

Create Comfort Intentionally

Comfort often happens by accident, yet today invites you to create it deliberately through small choices that help your body and mind feel more at ease.

This might look like adjusting your environment, choosing softer pacing, or allowing yourself a moment of quiet without distraction or explanation.

Intentional comfort is not indulgence, but a way of signaling safety and presence to yourself during the day.

Hold this truth gently today:
 I am allowed to create comfort.

FEBRUARY 10

Let Yourself Be Human

There is pressure to appear composed and capable at all times, yet today invites you to release that expectation and allow yourself to be fully human.

Being human means experiencing fatigue, uncertainty, emotion, and learning as you go, without needing to justify these experiences.

Notice moments when you expect yourself to operate without limits, and gently remind yourself that humanity includes rest and imperfection.

Carry this thought with you today:
I am allowed to be human.

FEBRUARY 11

Give Yourself Credit

It is easy to move past your own efforts without acknowledgment, yet today invites you to pause and recognize what you have already done.

Giving yourself credit does not require comparison or exaggeration, only honest recognition of effort, growth, or persistence.

Take a moment today to notice something you handled with care, even if it feels small or ordinary.

As the day continues, remember:
My efforts deserve recognition.

FEBRUARY 12

Slow Racing Thoughts

Racing thoughts often signal overstimulation rather than urgency, and today invites you to notice when your mind begins to speed ahead of your body.

Slowing your thoughts does not require stopping them completely, but allowing space through breathing, grounding, or gentle focus.

Pause briefly today when your mind feels crowded, letting steadiness return without force.

Let this reminder guide you:
I allow my thoughts to slow.

FEBRUARY 13

Welcome Gentle Pleasure

Pleasure does not need to be intense or dramatic to be meaningful, and today invites you to notice gentle moments of enjoyment without questioning or dismissing them.

Gentle pleasure may appear through warmth, comfort, beauty, or familiarity, asking only to be acknowledged.

Allow yourself to linger briefly with something pleasant today, letting it nourish you without turning it into a task.

Carry this thought forward:
I welcome gentle pleasure.

FEBRUARY 14

Care for Your Body Kindly

Your body carries you through every day, and today invites you to approach it with kindness rather than criticism or neglect.

Caring for your body kindly means listening to its signals and responding with patience, whether that involves rest, movement, nourishment, or softness.

Notice one way today to treat your body with respect rather than judgment, allowing care to feel supportive rather than corrective.

As you move on, remember:
I care for my body with kindness.

FEBRUARY 15

Replace Pressure With Patience

Pressure often creates the feeling that you must move faster or do more to be worthy of rest or ease, and today invites you to notice where patience might offer greater support.

Replacing pressure with patience does not mean giving up on growth, but allowing progress to unfold without constant urgency or self-surveillance.

Pause today when you feel rushed or tense, and consciously choose a slower, steadier response that gives your body room to settle.

As you continue through the day, let this reminder guide you:
 I choose patience over pressure.

FEBRUARY 16

Respect Emotional Boundaries

Emotional boundaries help you stay connected to yourself without absorbing more than you can reasonably hold, and today invites you to notice where yours may need attention.

Respecting emotional boundaries means allowing yourself to step back, pause conversations, or limit exposure without guilt or justification.

Notice how your body responds when you protect your emotional space, often feeling lighter or more grounded as a result.

Carry this truth gently today:
 My emotional boundaries matter.

FEBRUARY 17

Release Comparison Softly

Comparison can quietly undermine self-compassion, and today invites you to notice when you measure yourself against others without meaning to.

Releasing comparison does not require denying differences, but gently redirecting attention back to your own experience and pace.

When comparison arises today, soften your focus and remind yourself that your path does not need validation through contrast.

Hold this reminder close:
I release comparison with care.

FEBRUARY 18

Receive Care Freely

Receiving care can feel uncomfortable when you are used to giving or managing on your own, yet today invites you to allow support without resistance.

Receiving care does not create obligation or weakness, but acknowledges your shared humanity and your right to be supported.

Notice how it feels today to accept help, kindness, or understanding without immediately deflecting or minimizing it.

As you move forward, remember:
I allow myself to receive care.

FEBRUARY 19

Check In With Yourself

Daily life can pull attention outward, and today invites you to return inward with a brief, honest check-in.

Checking in does not require solving anything, but simply noticing how you feel physically and emotionally in this moment.

Allow this awareness to guide your next choice, even if the adjustment is small or internal.

Let this thought accompany you:
 I check in with myself.

FEBRUARY 20

Sit With What Arises

There is often an impulse to distract or fix uncomfortable feelings, yet today invites you to stay present with whatever arises without rushing it away.

Sitting with emotions does not mean intensifying them, but allowing them space to move and soften naturally.

Notice how your body responds when you stop resisting what you feel, often settling more than expected.

Carry this reminder gently:
I can sit with my experience.

FEBRUARY 21

Be Patient With Growth

Growth rarely follows a straight or predictable line, and today invites you to allow your process to unfold without constant evaluation.

Being patient with growth means trusting that effort accumulates even when results are not immediately visible.

Pause today to acknowledge where you are without rushing toward where you think you should be.

As the day continues, remember:
 I trust my pace of growth.

FEBRUARY 22

Offer Yourself Understanding

Understanding yourself requires slowing down enough to listen without immediately correcting or criticizing what you find, and today invites you to approach yourself with that patience.

Offering understanding means acknowledging that your reactions, emotions, and needs come from somewhere meaningful, even when they feel inconvenient or confusing.

Pause today when something feels difficult and ask what understanding might look like instead of judgment or dismissal.

Let this reminder guide you gently:
I meet myself with understanding.

FEBRUARY 23

Breathe Through Emotions

Emotions often move through the body before the mind can make sense of them, and today invites you to use your breath as a steady anchor when feelings arise.

Breathing through emotions does not mean controlling them, but allowing your breath to create space so they can pass without overwhelming you.

When you notice emotional intensity today, slow your breathing slightly and let your body respond with softness.

Carry this thought with you:
My breath supports me through emotion.

FEBRUARY 24

Appreciate Your Resilience

Resilience is often built quietly through moments you did not think you could handle, yet here you are, continuing forward with care and effort.

Today invites you to notice the ways you have adapted, endured, and learned, even when recognition was absent or delayed.

Allow yourself to acknowledge your resilience without minimizing it or comparing it to others' experiences.

Hold this reminder close:
I honor my resilience.

FEBRUARY 25

End the Month Kindly

As February begins to close, today invites you to look back on the month with kindness rather than evaluation or critique.

Ending the month kindly means acknowledging effort, learning, and presence without focusing solely on what you wish had been different.

Take a brief moment today to appreciate the care you offered yourself, even if it felt inconsistent or subtle.

Let this thought accompany you:
I end this month with kindness.

FEBRUARY 26

Carry Compassion Forward

Compassion is not meant to stay contained within a single moment or month, and today invites you to notice how it can continue alongside you.

Carrying compassion forward means allowing gentleness to inform your choices, especially when things feel unfinished or uncertain.

Pause today to consider how compassion might guide you into the days ahead without adding pressure.

Hold this reminder gently:
I carry compassion with me.

FEBRUARY 27

Rest in Self-Acceptance

Self-acceptance is not a destination to reach, but a place to rest when striving becomes heavy or unnecessary.

Today invites you to pause the effort to improve or correct yourself and simply allow who you are to be enough in this moment.

Notice how your body responds when acceptance replaces tension, even briefly.

Carry this truth with you:
 I rest in self-acceptance.

FEBRUARY 28

Close With Care

Closing a chapter does not require finality or certainty, but it does offer a moment to pause and acknowledge where you are before moving on.

Today invites you to close this month gently, without rushing ahead or leaving parts of yourself behind.

Allow yourself to feel the steadiness that comes from care practiced over time, even in small ways.

As you step forward, remember:
I move ahead with care.

MARCH

Clarity & Growth

March brings a subtle shift in energy, inviting you to see more clearly where you are and where you are being guided, without pressure to rush forward or have everything resolved.

This month focuses on clearing mental clutter, reconnecting with what matters, and allowing growth to happen through awareness rather than force or constant self-correction.

Clarity is not about having all the answers, but about creating enough space to recognize what feels aligned, meaningful, and steady beneath the noise of daily life.

As you move through March, allow understanding to deepen naturally, trusting that growth follows when you see yourself and your choices with honesty and care.

MARCH 1

Clarify What Matters Most

Life can easily become filled with competing priorities and expectations, and today invites you to pause long enough to notice what truly holds meaning for you beneath urgency, noise, and external demands.

Clarifying what matters most does not require final answers or dramatic decisions, but instead asks you to gently observe where your energy, attention, and sense of purpose naturally return over time.

As you move through the day, notice moments when something feels aligned or misaligned, allowing that awareness to guide your choices without forcing immediate change or explanation.

Clarity grows when you give yourself permission to focus on what feels essential rather than reacting to everything that asks for your attention.

MARCH 2

Reduce Mental Noise

The mind can easily become crowded with information, expectations, and unfinished thoughts, and today invites you to notice how much mental noise you are carrying without questioning whether it all deserves your attention.

Reducing mental noise does not mean forcing thoughts to stop, but gently creating space by stepping back from what feels repetitive, overwhelming, or unnecessary in this moment.

As you move through the day, notice when your attention feels scattered, and allow yourself to pause, breathe, or simplify without trying to solve everything at once.

Clarity often emerges not from effort or analysis, but from allowing enough quiet for what matters to rise naturally.

MARCH 3

Choose Focus Today

Attention is often pulled in many directions without your consent, and today invites you to gently choose where your focus rests rather than allowing it to scatter throughout the day.

Choosing focus does not require intensity or control, but a quiet commitment to stay present with what feels most important in this moment.

As you move through your day, notice when distractions arise, and softly return your attention without frustration or self-criticism.

Focus becomes steadier when it is guided by intention rather than force.

MARCH 4

Revisit Core Values

Your core values quietly shape your choices and reactions, even when they are not consciously acknowledged, and today invites you to reconnect with what truly matters beneath routine and obligation.

Revisiting your values does not require redefining them, but simply remembering what feels meaningful, grounding, and consistent over time.

Notice moments today when your actions feel aligned or misaligned, allowing that awareness to guide your decisions gently.

Clarity deepens when your choices reflect what you value most.

MARCH 5

Make One Intentional Choice

Life is shaped by many small choices made each day, and today invites you to bring awareness to just one decision instead of moving entirely on habit.

An intentional choice does not need to be dramatic, but it does benefit from a brief pause that allows you to act with presence rather than pressure.

As you move through the day, notice how it feels to choose deliberately, even in ordinary situations.

Small intentional choices create a quiet sense of direction over time.

MARCH 6

Reconnect With Curiosity

Curiosity has a way of softening rigidity and opening space where things have begun to feel fixed or routine. Today invites you to notice where you may have replaced interest with assumption. Reconnecting with curiosity allows experience to feel lighter and more alive.

Approaching life with curiosity does not mean searching for answers or solutions. It simply means allowing yourself to wonder without needing immediate clarity. This openness creates room for insight without pressure.

As you move through the day, notice moments when curiosity arises naturally. Let yourself linger there without rushing forward. Curiosity often guides growth quietly.

MARCH 7

Ask Honest Questions

Honest questions can bring clarity when certainty feels out of reach. Today invites you to ask what is true for you without shaping the answer in advance. Allow the question itself to be enough.

Asking honest questions requires gentleness rather than urgency. It means admitting when you do not fully understand what you are feeling or wanting. This honesty creates space for insight to emerge naturally.

Notice what questions surface today without forcing responses. Let them remain open if they need time. Clarity often grows from patience with uncertainty.

MARCH 8

Learn Without Pressure

Learning often becomes heavy when it is tied to comparison or expectation. Today invites you to approach learning as something that unfolds gradually rather than something to complete or master. This shift allows understanding to feel supportive instead of demanding.

Learning without pressure means allowing yourself to be a beginner again. It means noticing insights as they arrive instead of measuring progress. This approach creates steadiness rather than strain.

As you move through the day, notice moments of learning that happen quietly. Let them register without evaluation. Growth deepens when learning feels safe.

MARCH 9

Notice Growth Already Happening

Growth does not always announce itself clearly or dramatically. Today invites you to notice changes that may already be unfolding beneath the surface. These shifts often appear in how you respond rather than what you accomplish.

Notice moments when something feels easier than it once did. Pay attention to emotional responses that feel calmer or more grounded. These are signs of growth worth acknowledging.

As you move through the day, allow yourself to recognize progress without minimizing it. Let awareness replace self-judgment. Growth becomes clearer when you slow down enough to see it.

MARCH 10

Welcome Fresh Perspective

A fresh perspective can quietly change how you experience familiar situations. Today invites you to look again rather than assume you already know what something means. Openness creates room for clarity to shift.

Welcoming a new perspective does not require abandoning what you believe. It simply means allowing understanding to expand or adjust. This flexibility supports growth without conflict.

Notice moments today when your view softens or widens. Let curiosity guide you instead of certainty. Perspective often changes when you allow yourself to see again.

MARCH 11

Adjust Expectations Thoughtfully

Expectations often shape how you experience your day before anything actually happens. Today invites you to notice which expectations feel supportive and which quietly create pressure. Thoughtful adjustment begins with awareness rather than criticism.

Adjusting expectations does not mean lowering standards or giving up on what matters. It means aligning what you expect with your current energy, capacity, and circumstances. This alignment allows effort to feel steadier and more humane.

As you move through the day, notice moments when expectations feel heavy or unrealistic. Allow yourself to soften them where possible without guilt or explanation. Small adjustments can create noticeable relief.

When expectations are thoughtful rather than rigid, your experience becomes more spacious. You give yourself permission to meet the day as it is rather than how you think it should be. Clarity often follows this gentler approach.

MARCH 12

Trust Inner Guidance

Inner guidance often speaks quietly through feelings, instincts, or repeated thoughts rather than clear instructions. Today invites you to notice those subtle signals without dismissing them as insignificant. Trust begins with listening.

Trusting inner guidance does not mean having absolute certainty or ignoring outside input. It means allowing your own sense of alignment to have a voice in your decisions. This balance supports clarity rather than confusion.

As you move through the day, notice moments when something feels right or wrong without obvious explanation. Allow yourself to pause and acknowledge those signals. Awareness strengthens trust over time.

Inner guidance grows clearer when you treat it with respect and patience. You do not need to act on every signal immediately. Simply noticing builds a stronger connection.

MARCH 13

Plant Seeds for Change

Change often begins quietly, long before results are visible or measurable. Today invites you to focus on beginnings rather than outcomes or timelines. Small intentions can carry more power than dramatic efforts.

Planting seeds for change means choosing actions that feel aligned, even when progress feels slow. It allows you to trust that growth happens beneath the surface. Patience becomes part of the process.

As you move through the day, notice small actions that support the future you are moving toward. Let those actions be enough for now. Not every step needs immediate confirmation.

Growth responds best when it is allowed to unfold naturally. Seeds do not rush their own becoming. Your efforts are taking root.

MARCH 14

Release Unnecessary Obligations

Obligations can accumulate quietly until they begin to feel heavy or restrictive. Today invites you to notice which responsibilities truly require your energy and which persist out of habit or expectation. Awareness is the first step toward release.

Releasing unnecessary obligations does not mean avoiding responsibility. It means choosing where your time and energy are most meaningfully placed. This choice restores balance rather than creating loss.

As you move through the day, notice moments where saying yes feels draining. Allow yourself to question whether every obligation still fits. Space opens when pressure is reduced.

Letting go creates room for clarity and ease. You are allowed to choose intentionally. Not everything must be carried forward.

MARCH 15

Decide With Calm Confidence

Decisions often feel heavier when urgency or self-doubt takes the lead. Today invites you to approach choices with steadiness rather than pressure. Calm creates space for clarity.

Calm confidence does not require certainty or perfect information. It grows when you trust yourself enough to choose without rehearsing every possible outcome. This trust builds through practice.

As you move through the day, pause briefly before making decisions. Allow your body and breath to settle first. Clear choices often follow quiet moments.

Confidence strengthens when decisions feel grounded rather than rushed. You do not need to force assurance. Calm can guide you forward.

MARCH 16

Reclaim Mental Space

Mental space can become crowded without notice, filled with unfinished thoughts and constant stimulation. Today invites you to notice where your attention feels stretched or overwhelmed. Awareness creates the possibility of release.

Reclaiming mental space does not require solving everything at once. It means choosing what deserves attention now and what can wait. This choice brings relief rather than avoidance.

As you move through the day, notice moments when stepping back feels supportive. Allow yourself to disengage briefly from unnecessary mental effort. Space allows clarity to return.

A quieter mind often reveals what truly matters. You are allowed to rest from constant thinking. Mental space is a form of care.

MARCH 17

Focus on What's Controllable

Uncertainty can pull attention toward what lies beyond your control. Today invites you to gently redirect focus toward what remains within your influence. This shift creates steadiness.

Focusing on what's controllable does not deny uncertainty. It anchors you in actions, choices, and responses that are available right now. This grounding reduces unnecessary strain.

As you move through the day, notice where worry arises. Ask yourself what you can meaningfully address in this moment. Let that guide your energy.

Control is not about dominance, but about clarity. When focus narrows, calm often follows. You can move forward one grounded step at a time.

MARCH 18

Progress Over Perfection

Perfection often feels like safety, yet it can quietly prevent movement and learning. Today invites you to value progress instead of waiting for conditions to feel ideal. Forward motion matters more than flawless results.

Choosing progress allows you to stay engaged even when things feel unfinished or uncertain. It creates room for adjustment rather than self-criticism. This approach supports growth without unnecessary pressure.

As you move through the day, notice moments when you hesitate because something is not perfect. Allow yourself to continue anyway. Progress builds confidence through action.

Growth responds to consistency more than precision. Each step adds momentum. You are allowed to learn as you go.

MARCH 19

Reflect on Recent Lessons

Life is constantly offering lessons, though they are easy to miss when days feel busy or demanding. Today invites you to pause and notice what recent experiences have been teaching you. Reflection turns experience into understanding.

Reflecting does not require judgment or analysis. It simply asks you to observe patterns, insights, or changes that have emerged. Awareness brings clarity without pressure.

As you move through the day, allow moments of insight to surface naturally. You do not need to act on them immediately. Let understanding settle in its own time.

Lessons often become clearer when you give them space. Reflection strengthens awareness. Clarity grows through noticing.

MARCH 20

Invite Curiosity Into Routine

Routine can begin to feel dull when it runs on autopilot. Today invites you to bring curiosity into familiar moments. Small shifts in attention can change how you experience the ordinary.

Inviting curiosity does not mean disrupting your day. It means noticing details, sensations, or patterns you usually overlook. Curiosity refreshes without requiring change.

As you move through routine tasks, allow yourself to observe without judgment. Let interest replace assumption. Familiar moments can feel new again.

Curiosity keeps experience flexible. It supports engagement without effort. Growth often appears in small observations.

MARCH 21

Simplify One Commitment

Commitments can quietly multiply until they begin to feel heavy. Today invites you to look at one obligation and consider whether it still fits your priorities and energy. Simplification creates space.

Simplifying does not mean abandoning responsibility. It means choosing what deserves your attention right now. This choice restores balance rather than reducing care.

As you move through the day, notice which commitments feel supportive and which feel draining. Allow yourself to adjust one without guilt. Small changes can bring relief.

Simplicity often clarifies direction. Less pressure allows focus. You are allowed to choose thoughtfully.

MARCH 22

Strengthen Self-Awareness

Self-awareness grows when you pause long enough to notice what is happening within you. Today invites you to observe thoughts, emotions, and physical sensations as they arise. Awareness creates clarity.

Strengthening self-awareness does not mean constant analysis. It means noticing patterns without rushing to change them. This gentle attention builds understanding.

As you move through the day, notice how your body responds to situations before your mind reacts. Let that information guide your pace or choices. Presence deepens insight.

Self-awareness supports steady growth. It creates a stronger relationship with yourself. Clarity develops through consistent noticing.

MARCH 23

Move Forward Clearly

Clarity does not always arrive as certainty, but often as a quiet sense of direction. Today invites you to notice what feels steady enough to guide your next step. You do not need to see the entire path.

Moving forward clearly means trusting what feels aligned in this moment. It allows you to act without forcing confidence or demanding reassurance. Small clarity is still clarity.

As you move through the day, notice when decisions feel calm rather than urgent. Let that feeling guide your pace and choices. Clarity often feels grounded, not loud.

Moving forward clearly is about responsiveness, not control. You adjust as you learn more. Direction strengthens through presence.

MARCH 24

Close the Month Mindfully

As the month nears its end, today invites you to slow down and take notice. Reflection allows experience to settle rather than rush past. Mindful closure creates continuity.

Closing the month mindfully does not require evaluation or judgment. It simply asks you to acknowledge what this period has offered. Awareness replaces critique.

As you move through the day, notice moments of growth, effort, or learning. Allow them to be seen without measuring their value. Recognition itself is meaningful.

Mindful endings prepare you for thoughtful beginnings. They allow you to carry insight forward. Nothing needs to be rushed.

MARCH 25

Trust Your Direction

Trusting your direction does not mean having certainty about outcomes. Today invites you to honor the choices you are making with the understanding you currently have. Trust grows through consistency.

Doubt may still appear, but it does not need to lead. Allow yourself to move forward even when clarity feels incomplete. Direction often strengthens after action.

As you move through the day, notice when your choices feel aligned rather than approved. Let that alignment matter. Trust develops through lived experience.

Direction is not fixed; it adapts as you do. Trust allows flexibility without self-abandonment. Growth follows engagement.

MARCH 26

Grow Without Rushing

Growth can become strained when it is rushed or forced. Today invites you to allow progress to unfold at a pace that feels sustainable. Patience supports depth.

Growing without rushing means releasing the belief that visible results must appear quickly. It allows learning and integration to happen fully. Slow growth often lasts longer.

As you move through the day, notice moments when slowing down feels supportive. Let yourself take the time you need. Growth does not need pressure to continue.

Steady progress builds resilience. It honors your capacity. You are allowed to grow at your own pace.

MARCH 27

Honor Small Progress

Small progress is easy to overlook when attention stays fixed on larger goals. Today invites you to notice movement that happens quietly and consistently. Recognition builds momentum.

Honoring small progress means acknowledging effort without minimizing it. It allows you to see growth even when outcomes feel incomplete. Awareness strengthens confidence.

As you move through the day, notice one small way you have moved forward. Let that recognition be enough. Progress accumulates over time.

Honoring progress supports continuation. It reinforces trust in yourself. Growth becomes easier to sustain.

MARCH 28

Honor Small Progress

Small progress often goes unnoticed when attention stays fixed on what remains undone. Today invites you to slow down and recognize movement that has already taken place. Acknowledgment strengthens momentum.

Honoring small progress means valuing effort, consistency, and awareness even when results feel incomplete. It allows you to see growth without demanding perfection. This recognition builds confidence quietly.

As you move through the day, notice one small step you have taken recently. Let yourself appreciate it without minimizing its importance. Progress accumulates through moments like these.

Small progress deserves respect. It reflects commitment and presence. Growth continues through steady acknowledgment.

MARCH 29

Grow Without Rushing

Growth can lose its meaning when it is rushed or forced. Today invites you to notice where patience might serve you better than urgency. Slowing down often allows understanding to deepen.

Growing without rushing means trusting your process instead of comparing it to imagined timelines. It allows learning to settle rather than skim the surface. Depth develops through time.

As you move through the day, notice moments when you feel pressured to move faster than feels natural. Allow yourself to choose steadiness instead. Growth does not require speed.

Progress unfolds at its own pace. You are allowed to take the time you need. Sustainable growth honors capacity.

MARCH 30

Trust Your Direction

Trusting your direction does not require certainty about outcomes. Today invites you to honor the path you are already walking. Trust develops through continued engagement.

Doubt may still appear, but it does not need to lead your choices. Direction becomes clearer when you stay present with what feels aligned. Confidence grows through action.

As you move through the day, notice moments when your choices feel steady rather than approved. Let alignment matter more than reassurance. Direction strengthens through lived experience.

Trust allows flexibility without self-abandonment. You are permitted to adjust as you learn. Growth follows honest movement.

MARCH 31

Close the Month Mindfully

As March comes to an end, today invites you to pause rather than rush forward. Mindful closure allows experiences to settle instead of being carried unfinished into the next chapter. Reflection brings integration.

Closing the month mindfully does not require evaluation or judgment. It simply asks you to notice what has shifted, clarified, or softened. Awareness replaces critique.

As you move through the day, allow yourself to acknowledge effort, insight, and presence. Let this recognition feel complete without needing improvement. Ending gently prepares you to begin again.

Mindful endings support thoughtful beginnings. You carry clarity forward with you. Nothing needs to be forced.

APRIL

Renewal & Energy

April brings a natural sense of renewal, inviting you to reawaken gently rather than forcing yourself into motion or change. This month focuses on restoring energy through attention, rhythm, and kindness toward your body and mind. Renewal here is not about doing more, but about reconnecting with what already supports vitality.

Energy returns most sustainably when it is respected rather than demanded. April encourages you to notice where life feels lighter, more spacious, or quietly motivating. Growth unfolds when you allow renewal to feel simple.

As you move through this month, let energy rise gradually. Trust that steadiness creates strength. Renewal begins with listening.

APRIL 1

Wake Your Body Gently

The way you begin your day often shapes how your body carries energy forward. Today invites you to wake yourself gently rather than rushing into movement or expectation. Soft beginnings support steadier momentum.

Waking gently means noticing your body before asking it to perform. It allows muscles, breath, and awareness to arrive together. This care builds trust with yourself.

As you move through the morning, notice how gentleness affects your energy. Allow yourself to move slowly if needed. Energy responds well to patience.

Gentle waking sets a supportive tone. It reminds you that energy does not need force. Renewal begins quietly.

APRIL 2

Invite Fresh Energy

Fresh energy often arrives when you make space for it rather than chasing it. Today invites you to notice where openness allows vitality to return naturally. Invitation creates flow.

Inviting energy does not require intensity or motivation. It begins with small shifts in attention, breath, or movement. These subtle changes support renewal.

As you move through the day, notice moments when energy feels lighter or clearer. Allow those moments to guide your pace. Energy grows through awareness.

Fresh energy responds to permission. You do not need to push. Openness is enough.

APRIL 3

Step Outside Intentionally

Stepping outside can quietly reset your energy and perspective. Today invites you to do so with intention rather than distraction. Presence deepens restoration.

Being outside does not require effort or productivity. It simply asks you to notice light, air, and movement. These elements support balance naturally.

As you spend time outdoors, allow your senses to engage fully. Let your body respond without analysis. Nature restores without instruction.

Intentional time outside refreshes energy. It grounds awareness. Renewal becomes accessible.

APRIL 4

Refresh Daily Rhythms

Daily rhythms shape how energy flows through your life. Today invites you to notice where routines feel supportive and where they feel draining. Awareness opens possibility.

Refreshing rhythms does not mean changing everything at once. It means making small adjustments that restore balance. These shifts build sustainability.

As you move through the day, notice when your energy rises or dips. Let that information guide gentle changes. Rhythm supports renewal.

Balanced rhythms conserve energy. They create steadiness. Renewal follows consistency.

APRIL 5

Welcome Lightness Today

Lightness often appears when pressure eases. Today invites you to notice where you can soften effort and allow ease. Lightness supports vitality.

Welcoming lightness does not mean avoiding responsibility. It means releasing unnecessary heaviness in how you approach your day. This shift restores energy.

As you move through the day, notice moments when things feel less weighted. Allow yourself to remain there briefly. Ease is nourishing.

Lightness refreshes energy naturally. It creates space to breathe. Renewal feels simpler.

APRIL 6

Stretch Without Expectations

Stretching can become another task when it is tied to outcomes or performance, and today invites you to approach movement as a way of listening rather than achieving. This gentle attention allows your body to respond honestly. Ease replaces pressure.

Stretching without expectations means noticing sensation without trying to improve or correct it. It allows movement to feel exploratory rather than demanding. This approach supports energy rather than draining it.

As you move your body today, notice where it feels open and where it resists. Allow each sensation to exist without judgment. Awareness guides care.

Gentle stretching restores connection. It reminds you that your body does not need to be fixed. Renewal grows through acceptance.

APRIL 7

Breathe in Possibility

Breath has the ability to quietly shift how energy moves through your body. Today invites you to breathe with awareness rather than habit. Attention creates openness.

Breathing in possibility does not mean forcing optimism. It means allowing each breath to feel spacious and supportive. This openness refreshes energy naturally.

As you move through the day, notice moments when your breath becomes shallow or tense. Allow yourself to slow it gently. Breath restores balance.

Possibility often enters through simple awareness. Breath creates space. Renewal begins internally.

APRIL 8

Let Nature Restore You

Nature offers restoration without asking for effort or understanding. Today invites you to allow natural surroundings to support your energy. Presence deepens restoration.

Letting nature restore you means receiving rather than doing. It asks only that you notice light, sound, air, or movement. These elements calm and renew.

As you spend time outdoors, allow your senses to guide attention. Let your body respond without analysis. Restoration happens quietly.

Nature restores without instruction. It reminds you how to slow down. Renewal feels effortless.

APRIL 9

Move in Enjoyable Ways

Movement becomes energizing when it is enjoyable rather than obligatory. Today invites you to notice what kinds of movement feel supportive and pleasant. Enjoyment sustains vitality.

Moving in enjoyable ways means listening to preference instead of expectation. It allows your body to guide pace and intensity. This respect builds energy.

As you move today, notice how enjoyment affects motivation. Allow pleasure to inform duration and effort. Energy responds to enjoyment.

Enjoyable movement feels nourishing. It restores connection with your body. Renewal follows pleasure.

APRIL 10

Refresh Your Environment

Your surroundings quietly influence how your energy feels throughout the day. Today invites you to notice whether your environment supports or drains you. Awareness opens choice.

Refreshing your environment does not require major changes. Small adjustments can restore clarity and ease. These shifts affect energy more than expected.

As you move through your space, notice what feels heavy or stagnant. Allow yourself to refresh one small area. Environment shapes vitality.

A refreshed environment supports focus. It allows energy to circulate. Renewal becomes tangible.

APRIL 11

Reignite Motivation Slowly

Motivation often fades when it is forced or expected to appear all at once. Today invites you to approach motivation as something that can be rekindled gradually rather than demanded. Slowness allows energy to return naturally.

Reigniting motivation slowly means paying attention to small sparks of interest or willingness. It allows you to build momentum without pressure or comparison. This approach supports sustainable energy.

As you move through the day, notice moments when curiosity or engagement arises. Let those moments guide your actions gently. Motivation grows through patience.

Slow motivation feels steadier. It respects your current capacity. Renewal unfolds without strain.

APRIL 12

Nourish Energy Wisely

Energy is influenced by how you care for yourself throughout the day. Today invites you to notice which habits support vitality and which quietly drain it. Awareness creates balance.

Nourishing energy wisely means choosing what replenishes rather than what merely distracts. It allows you to respond thoughtfully to your body's signals. This care preserves strength.

As you move through the day, notice how food, rest, and stimulation affect your energy. Allow yourself to adjust without guilt. Wise nourishment sustains momentum.

Balanced care supports lasting energy. It prevents depletion. Renewal becomes consistent.

APRIL 13

Balance Action With Rest

Action and rest work best when they support each other. Today invites you to notice whether your day includes space for both movement and pause. Balance restores flow.

Balancing action with rest does not mean equal time for each. It means honoring when your body needs activity and when it needs stillness. This awareness prevents burnout.

As you move through the day, notice signs of fatigue or restlessness. Allow yourself to respond appropriately. Balance supports resilience.

Rest enhances action. Action feels lighter with rest. Renewal depends on both.

APRIL 14

Start the Day Curious

The way you begin the day influences how energy unfolds. Today invites you to start with curiosity rather than assumption or urgency. Openness refreshes awareness.

Starting the day curious means noticing how you feel without immediately labeling or judging it. It allows experience to unfold naturally. Curiosity keeps energy flexible.

As your day begins, notice what captures your interest. Allow curiosity to guide attention briefly. Engagement grows from openness.

Curiosity invites presence. Presence supports energy. Renewal follows awareness.

APRIL 15

Release Stagnant Patterns

Stagnant patterns can quietly drain energy when they repeat without reflection. Today invites you to notice habits or routines that no longer feel supportive. Awareness creates possibility.

Releasing stagnant patterns does not require immediate change. It begins with acknowledging what feels stuck or outdated. This recognition opens space.

As you move through the day, notice moments where you act automatically. Allow yourself to pause and choose differently if needed. Change begins gently.

Releasing stagnation restores flow. Energy responds to openness. Renewal becomes possible.

APRIL 16

Practice Energizing Rest

Rest can be energizing when it is intentional rather than reactive. Today invites you to notice how different kinds of rest affect your body and mind. Not all rest looks the same.

Practicing energizing rest means choosing pauses that genuinely restore you. It may involve stillness, quiet attention, or stepping away from stimulation. This kind of rest supports vitality.

As you move through the day, notice moments when rest feels refreshing rather than numbing. Allow yourself to choose that kind of pause. Energy returns through thoughtful rest.

Energizing rest creates balance. It supports clarity and strength. Renewal becomes sustainable.

APRIL 17

Reconnect With Vitality

Vitality is often present even when energy feels low. Today invites you to notice where aliveness still exists within you. Awareness helps it surface.

Reconnecting with vitality does not require dramatic change. It begins by noticing moments of engagement, warmth, or interest. These signals point toward renewal.

As you move through the day, notice what brings a sense of liveliness. Allow yourself to stay with those moments briefly. Vitality grows through attention.

Vitality responds to care. It strengthens through recognition. Renewal feels more accessible.

APRIL 18

Do Something Playful

Playfulness can refresh energy in ways effort cannot. Today invites you to allow space for lightness and enjoyment. Play restores balance.

Doing something playful does not require planning or justification. It means allowing yourself to engage in something simply because it feels pleasant. This permission supports vitality.

As you move through the day, notice moments when playfulness feels possible. Let yourself follow that impulse briefly. Energy responds to joy.

Play reconnects you with ease. It softens pressure. Renewal feels lighter.

APRIL 19

Trust Renewing Strength

Strength often rebuilds quietly rather than dramatically. Today invites you to trust that renewal is happening even when progress feels subtle. Patience supports recovery.

Trusting renewing strength means allowing your body and mind time to restore. It means releasing the urge to test or prove your energy. This trust prevents strain.

As you move through the day, notice signs of steadiness returning. Allow those signs to reassure you. Strength grows through consistency.

Renewal strengthens resilience. It builds quietly. Trust supports endurance.

APRIL 20

Restore What Feels Drained

Some areas of your life may feel more depleted than others. Today invites you to notice what feels drained without judgment. Awareness guides care.

Restoring what feels drained does not require addressing everything at once. It begins with choosing one area to support gently. Small care creates relief.

As you move through the day, notice where energy feels thin. Allow yourself to offer replenishment rather than pressure. Restoration begins with attention.

Care restores balance. Energy responds to kindness. Renewal becomes possible.

APRIL 21

Allow Gentle Momentum

Momentum builds most naturally when it is allowed to grow rather than pushed into existence. Today invites you to notice where movement already feels possible and to support it gently. Ease creates continuity.

Allowing gentle momentum means respecting your current pace instead of comparing it to expectations or past rhythms. It allows progress to feel steady rather than strained. This approach sustains energy.

As you move through the day, notice moments when actions flow with less resistance. Let yourself continue at that pace without forcing more. Momentum responds to patience.

Gentle momentum supports endurance. It honors your capacity. Renewal unfolds gradually.

APRIL 22

Choose Sustainable Energy

Energy is most supportive when it can be maintained over time. Today invites you to notice whether your actions are replenishing or depleting you. Sustainability creates balance.

Choosing sustainable energy means favoring habits and rhythms that support you consistently. It allows you to work with your energy rather than against it. This choice prevents burnout.

As you move through the day, notice when something feels energizing but draining afterward. Allow yourself to adjust toward steadiness. Energy thrives on sustainability.

Sustainable energy feels reliable. It supports clarity and focus. Renewal becomes lasting.

APRIL 23

End the Month Refreshed

As the month begins to draw toward its close, today invites you to notice how your energy feels now compared to earlier weeks. Reflection allows renewal to settle. Awareness replaces urgency.

Ending the month refreshed does not require constant productivity or visible achievement. It means acknowledging restoration wherever it has occurred. Recognition deepens renewal.

As you move through the day, notice moments of ease or clarity. Allow yourself to appreciate them without analysis. Refreshment grows through acknowledgment.

Gentle endings support continuity. They prepare you for what comes next. Renewal carries forward.

APRIL 24

Carry Renewal Forward

Renewal is most meaningful when it continues beyond a single moment or month. Today invites you to notice what practices or attitudes you want to carry forward. Continuity sustains energy.

Carrying renewal forward does not mean maintaining intensity. It means staying attentive to what supports balance and vitality. Small choices keep renewal alive.

As you move through the day, notice which habits feel worth continuing. Allow yourself to commit gently rather than rigidly. Renewal responds to care.

Sustained renewal feels flexible. It adapts with you. Energy remains supported.

APRIL 25

Appreciate Reawakened Energy

Reawakened energy often appears quietly, without announcement. Today invites you to notice and appreciate any return of motivation, clarity, or physical vitality. Appreciation strengthens awareness.

Appreciating energy does not mean clinging to it or fearing its loss. It means recognizing its presence without pressure. This acknowledgment supports balance.

As you move through the day, notice moments when energy feels lighter or more available. Allow yourself to register those moments fully. Awareness deepens renewal.

Appreciation reinforces vitality. It builds trust in your capacity. Renewal feels acknowledged.

APRIL 26

Honor the Body's Signals

Your body communicates its needs constantly, often before your mind has time to interpret them. Today invites you to notice physical sensations, shifts in energy, or moments of discomfort without dismissing or overriding them. Listening creates alignment.

Honoring the body's signals does not mean reacting immediately to every sensation. It means acknowledging what your body is communicating and allowing that information to guide your choices gently. Respect builds trust.

As you move through the day, notice when your body asks for rest, movement, or nourishment. Allow yourself to respond with care rather than resistance. Attention supports balance.

The body offers wisdom through sensation. When you listen, energy stabilizes. Renewal deepens through respect.

APRIL 27

Let Renewal Be Simple

Renewal does not need to be elaborate or demanding to be effective. Today invites you to notice how simplicity can restore energy more fully than complexity. Ease supports clarity.

Letting renewal be simple means releasing the idea that you must do more to feel better. It allows small, accessible actions to carry value. Simplicity reduces strain.

As you move through the day, notice where simplicity feels supportive. Allow yourself to choose the easier path without guilt. Energy responds to gentleness.

Simple renewal is sustainable. It fits into daily life. Vitality grows quietly.

APRIL 28

Stay Open to Change

Change often unfolds gradually, asking for openness rather than certainty. Today invites you to remain receptive to shifts in energy, perspective, or direction. Openness creates movement.

Staying open to change does not require constant adjustment. It means allowing possibilities to exist without resistance. This flexibility supports renewal.

As you move through the day, notice moments when change feels uncomfortable or unfamiliar. Allow curiosity to soften that response. Openness eases transition.

Change becomes less threatening when it is welcomed gently. Energy adapts more easily. Renewal continues through flexibility.

APRIL 29

Pause Before Pushing

The urge to push forward can arise when energy feels uneven or uncertain. Today invites you to pause before applying pressure to yourself or your body. Awareness prevents strain.

Pausing before pushing allows you to assess whether effort is truly needed or if rest would be more supportive. This pause creates choice. Balance follows awareness.

As you move through the day, notice moments when urgency appears. Allow yourself to slow briefly before responding. Pausing preserves energy.

Pressure often drains more than it delivers. Pauses restore perspective. Renewal benefits from restraint.

APRIL 30

Welcome Ease

Ease can feel unfamiliar when effort has become habitual. Today invites you to notice where ease is available and to allow it without suspicion or resistance. Acceptance supports restoration.

Welcoming ease does not mean avoiding responsibility. It means releasing unnecessary tension in how you approach what you do. This shift conserves energy.

As you move through the day, notice moments when things flow without struggle. Allow yourself to remain there briefly. Ease replenishes vitality.

Ease creates space for balance. It reminds you that renewal does not require effort. The month closes with gentleness.

MAY

Confidence & Self-Trust

May invites a steady return to confidence that grows from familiarity with yourself rather than performance or approval. This month focuses on strengthening trust in your judgment, your pace, and your ability to choose wisely over time. Confidence here is grounded, lived, and quiet.

Self-trust develops through repetition, reflection, and honoring experience. It does not need to announce itself or prove anything to others. Growth feels calmer when confidence is internal.

As you move through May, allow confidence to feel supportive rather than demanding. Let trust deepen through consistency. Self-assurance grows through attention.

MAY 1

Trust Your Judgment

Your judgment is shaped by experience, reflection, and awareness, even when doubt attempts to override it. Today invites you to notice where you already know what feels right for you. Trust begins with acknowledgment.

Trusting your judgment does not require certainty or flawless outcomes. It means allowing your perspective to matter alongside external input. Balance strengthens confidence.

As you move through the day, notice moments when you hesitate despite clarity. Allow yourself to proceed thoughtfully anyway. Trust grows through use.

Confidence develops through lived decisions. Each choice reinforces self-trust. Judgment strengthens over time.

MAY 2

Speak With Quiet Confidence

Confidence does not need volume to be effective. Today invites you to express yourself calmly and clearly without over-explaining or seeking reassurance. Presence carries weight.

Speaking with quiet confidence means trusting your words as they are. It allows you to communicate without defending your right to be heard. This steadiness builds respect.

As you move through conversations today, notice when fewer words feel sufficient. Allow clarity to replace justification. Confidence settles naturally.

Quiet confidence feels grounded. It does not rush or impress. Self-trust speaks steadily.

MAY 3

Honor Personal Limits

Personal limits protect energy, focus, and well-being. Today invites you to notice where boundaries support your confidence rather than restrict it. Limits clarify priorities.

Honoring limits does not mean withdrawal or avoidance. It means choosing what you can offer without self-compromise. This choice builds trust with yourself.

As you move through the day, notice when limits feel necessary. Allow yourself to honor them without apology. Respect strengthens confidence.

Limits reinforce self-trust. They create stability. Confidence grows through self-respect.

MAY 4

Believe Your Inner Voice

Your inner voice often speaks through intuition, repetition, or quiet insistence. Today invites you to listen without dismissing or second-guessing its guidance. Attention deepens trust.

Believing your inner voice does not require ignoring external perspectives. It means allowing your own insight to carry weight. Balance supports clarity.

As you move through the day, notice moments when your inner voice feels consistent. Allow yourself to acknowledge it. Trust strengthens through recognition.

Inner guidance grows clearer when respected. Confidence responds to listening. Self-trust deepens naturally.

MAY 5

Practice Calm Decisions

Decisions often feel heavier when rushed or emotionally charged. Today invites you to approach choices with calm rather than urgency. Stillness supports clarity.

Practicing calm decisions means pausing long enough to feel grounded before acting. It allows your judgment to guide you rather than pressure. This steadiness builds confidence.

As you move through the day, notice moments when slowing your response feels supportive. Allow calm to inform your choices. Confidence follows clarity.

Calm decisions strengthen self-trust. They reduce regret and strain. Confidence grows through steadiness.

MAY 6

Choose Self-Respect

Self-respect shapes how you treat yourself long before others respond. Today invites you to notice whether your choices reflect care, honesty, and fairness toward yourself. Awareness strengthens dignity.

Choosing self-respect does not require confrontation or explanation. It means acting in ways that align with your values and limits. This alignment builds confidence quietly.

As you move through the day, notice moments when self-respect guides your decisions. Allow yourself to honor that guidance without hesitation. Confidence follows integrity.

Self-respect reinforces self-trust. It creates inner stability. Confidence grows through alignment.

MAY 7

Stand by Your Needs

Your needs provide important information about balance and well-being. Today invites you to acknowledge them without minimizing or justifying their existence. Recognition supports confidence.

Standing by your needs does not mean demanding or withdrawing. It means allowing your needs to matter alongside responsibilities and relationships. This balance strengthens trust.

As you move through the day, notice when your needs surface clearly. Allow yourself to respond with care rather than dismissal. Confidence grows through acknowledgment.

Honoring needs builds self-trust. It prevents resentment. Confidence becomes steadier.

MAY 8

Strengthen Inner Assurance

Inner assurance develops through consistency rather than external validation. Today invites you to notice where confidence already exists quietly within you. Awareness reinforces stability.

Strengthening inner assurance means relying less on approval and more on lived experience. It allows confidence to feel grounded instead of reactive. This shift builds resilience.

As you move through the day, notice moments when you feel sure without explanation. Allow that feeling to remain. Inner assurance deepens through presence.

Confidence rooted within lasts longer. It adapts without strain. Self-trust becomes reliable.

MAY 9

Release External Approval

Seeking approval can quietly influence decisions and diminish confidence. Today invites you to notice where approval-seeking shapes your choices. Awareness restores agency.

Releasing external approval does not mean disregarding others. It means allowing your values to guide you first. This shift strengthens self-trust.

As you move through the day, notice moments when you hesitate for fear of judgment. Allow yourself to proceed thoughtfully anyway. Confidence grows through independence.

Letting go of approval frees energy. It clarifies direction. Confidence becomes internal.

MAY 10

Act From Self-Trust

Action feels steadier when it comes from trust rather than doubt. Today invites you to notice where self-trust can guide your next step. Awareness supports confidence.

Acting from self-trust does not require certainty. It means choosing with honesty and allowing outcomes to inform learning. This approach reduces hesitation.

As you move through the day, notice when your actions feel aligned rather than approved. Let alignment matter most. Confidence strengthens through experience.

Self-trust grows through action. It reinforces belief in yourself. Confidence becomes lived.

MAY 11

Celebrate Small Wins

Small wins often pass unnoticed when attention stays fixed on what remains undone. Today invites you to pause and recognize progress that has already occurred. Acknowledgment strengthens confidence.

Celebrating small wins does not require exaggeration or comparison. It means allowing effort and follow-through to be seen and valued. This recognition builds momentum.

As you move through the day, notice one action you completed or handled well. Allow yourself to acknowledge it without minimizing its importance. Confidence grows through appreciation.

Small wins accumulate over time. They reinforce self-belief. Confidence becomes more grounded.

MAY 12

Claim Personal Space

Personal space supports clarity, focus, and emotional balance. Today invites you to notice whether you are allowing yourself enough room to think, feel, and respond honestly. Space strengthens self-trust.

Claiming personal space does not require withdrawal or explanation. It means honoring your need for boundaries, time, or quiet. This choice supports confidence.

As you move through the day, notice moments when space feels necessary. Allow yourself to create it gently. Confidence grows through self-respect.

Personal space restores balance. It protects energy. Self-trust deepens through care.

MAY 13

Choose Confidence Over Doubt

Doubt can surface even when experience supports you. Today invites you to notice when doubt speaks louder than evidence. Awareness creates choice.

Choosing confidence does not mean ignoring uncertainty. It means allowing your experience and values to guide you more than fear. This shift builds steadiness.

As you move through the day, notice moments when doubt pauses you unnecessarily. Allow yourself to move forward thoughtfully anyway. Confidence strengthens through action.

Confidence grows with use. It quiets doubt over time. Self-trust becomes familiar.

MAY 14

Listen to Your Wisdom

Wisdom often develops through lived experience rather than instruction. Today invites you to notice insights that have emerged from what you have already navigated. Attention deepens trust.

Listening to your wisdom means valuing what you have learned through trial, reflection, and adjustment. It allows your knowledge to guide choices calmly. This builds confidence.

As you move through the day, notice moments when your past experience offers clarity. Allow yourself to rely on it. Wisdom strengthens through acknowledgment.

Your wisdom is earned. It deserves respect. Confidence grows through recognition.

MAY 15

Practice Assertive Kindness

Kindness and assertiveness can coexist without conflict. Today invites you to notice where honesty and care can be expressed together. Balance strengthens confidence.

Practicing assertive kindness means communicating needs and boundaries clearly while remaining respectful. It allows you to stand firm without harshness. This approach supports trust.

As you move through the day, notice moments when you can speak honestly with warmth. Allow yourself to do so without apology. Confidence grows through clarity.

Assertive kindness reinforces self-respect. It builds trust with others and yourself. Confidence becomes steady.

MAY 16

Recognize Inner Strength

Inner strength often shows itself through persistence, adaptation, and quiet endurance rather than dramatic moments. Today invites you to notice the strength you have already demonstrated through challenges and change. Recognition builds confidence.

Recognizing inner strength does not require comparison or external validation. It means acknowledging how you have supported yourself through difficulty. This awareness reinforces trust.

As you move through the day, notice moments when resilience appears naturally. Allow yourself to acknowledge it without minimizing its significance. Confidence grows through recognition.

Inner strength develops over time. It remains steady beneath uncertainty. Self-trust deepens through awareness.

MAY 17

Move Forward Unapologetically

Moving forward unapologetically means honoring your choices without constant explanation or justification. Today invites you to notice where hesitation comes from fear of judgment rather than misalignment. Awareness restores confidence.

This approach does not require dismissing others' perspectives. It means allowing your values and judgment to guide you without retreating. Confidence strengthens through clarity.

As you move through the day, notice moments when you soften or pull back unnecessarily. Allow yourself to stand firm gently. Confidence grows through self-authorization.

Moving forward unapologetically feels grounded. It respects your autonomy. Self-trust becomes visible.

MAY 18

Trust Yourself Today

Trust is built through daily reinforcement rather than occasional certainty. Today invites you to trust yourself in small, ordinary moments. Consistency builds confidence.

Trusting yourself today does not require perfect outcomes. It means allowing your judgment to guide decisions without excessive second-guessing. This steadiness reduces strain.

As you move through the day, notice moments when trust feels natural. Allow yourself to act from that place. Confidence grows through repetition.

Daily trust compounds over time. It strengthens belief in yourself. Confidence becomes familiar.

MAY 19

Let Confidence Be Quiet

Confidence does not always need expression or display. Today invites you to allow confidence to exist internally without proving itself. Quiet strength is sufficient.

Letting confidence be quiet means trusting yourself without seeking affirmation. It allows assurance to feel calm rather than performative. This steadiness builds resilience.

As you move through the day, notice moments when quiet confidence supports your actions. Allow yourself to remain grounded without explanation. Confidence settles naturally.

Quiet confidence feels secure. It does not rush or compete. Self-trust deepens in silence.

MAY 20

Reaffirm Capabilities

Your capabilities have been shaped through learning, effort, and experience. Today invites you to acknowledge what you are capable of without exaggeration or doubt. Recognition supports confidence.

Reaffirming capabilities does not mean ignoring growth areas. It means honoring skills and strengths that already exist. This balance builds trust.

As you move through the day, notice tasks you handle competently. Allow yourself to acknowledge this without dismissal. Confidence grows through honesty.

Capabilities become clearer when recognized. They support self-trust. Confidence stabilizes through awareness.

MAY 21

Stay Grounded in Choice

Every day presents choices that shape how you experience yourself and the world around you. Today invites you to remain grounded in the awareness that you are choosing, even in small or familiar moments. This recognition strengthens confidence.

Staying grounded in choice means noticing that you have agency even when options feel limited. It allows you to respond thoughtfully rather than react automatically. This awareness builds steadiness.

As you move through the day, notice moments when you choose deliberately instead of by habit. Allow yourself to acknowledge that agency. Confidence grows through conscious choice.

Grounded choices reinforce self-trust. They create clarity and direction. Confidence becomes intentional.

MAY 22

Lead Yourself Kindly

Leadership begins with how you treat yourself internally. Today invites you to guide your thoughts, actions, and expectations with kindness rather than criticism. Compassion strengthens confidence.

Leading yourself kindly does not mean avoiding accountability. It means encouraging growth without harshness or impatience. This approach supports resilience.

As you move through the day, notice your internal tone when challenges arise. Allow yourself to respond with understanding. Confidence grows through supportive leadership.

Kind self-leadership builds trust. It creates emotional safety. Confidence becomes sustainable.

MAY 23

End the Month Empowered

As the month moves toward its close, today invites you to recognize the confidence you have been building steadily. Reflection allows empowerment to settle rather than rush past. Awareness reinforces strength.

Ending the month empowered does not require dramatic change or visible transformation. It means acknowledging growth in judgment, boundaries, and self-trust. Recognition matters.

As you move through the day, notice where you feel more grounded than before. Allow yourself to honor that shift. Empowerment grows through acknowledgment.

Empowered endings support continuity. They prepare you to carry confidence forward. Strength feels integrated.

MAY 24

Carry Confidence Gently

Confidence is most supportive when it is carried with ease rather than force. Today invites you to notice how gentleness allows confidence to remain steady and accessible. Softness supports strength.

Carrying confidence gently means trusting yourself without defensiveness or rigidity. It allows confidence to adapt as situations change. This flexibility builds resilience.

As you move through the day, notice moments when calm assurance guides your actions. Allow yourself to remain in that space. Confidence flows naturally.

Gentle confidence feels grounded. It does not need to prove itself. Self-trust deepens quietly.

MAY 25

Believe in Consistency

Consistency often builds confidence more reliably than intensity. Today invites you to notice how repeated effort and presence have supported your growth. Awareness reinforces belief.

Believing in consistency means trusting that steady action creates meaningful change. It allows patience to replace urgency. This perspective supports self-trust.

As you move through the day, notice where you have shown up consistently. Allow yourself to recognize that commitment. Confidence grows through repetition.

Consistency strengthens reliability. It builds trust in yourself. Confidence becomes durable.

MAY 26

Honor Earned Growth

Growth that has been earned through experience deserves recognition rather than dismissal. Today invites you to notice how much you have learned, adjusted, and strengthened over time. Acknowledgment builds confidence.

Honoring earned growth means valuing progress that came through effort, patience, and reflection. It allows you to respect your journey without comparison. This respect deepens self-trust.

As you move through the day, notice moments when your growth supports you naturally. Allow yourself to recognize it without minimizing its importance. Confidence grows through acknowledgment.

Earned growth creates stability. It reflects resilience and learning. Self-trust becomes grounded.

MAY 27

Stay True to Yourself

Staying true to yourself requires awareness of what feels aligned beneath expectations and noise. Today invites you to notice where authenticity supports confidence. Alignment strengthens trust.

Staying true does not mean resisting change or ignoring feedback. It means allowing your values to remain central as you adapt. This balance builds integrity.

As you move through the day, notice moments when choices reflect your true priorities. Allow yourself to honor those moments. Confidence grows through authenticity.

Authenticity reinforces self-trust. It provides clarity and direction. Confidence feels steady.

MAY 28

Walk Your Own Path

Your path is shaped by experience, values, and timing that are uniquely yours. Today invites you to notice where comparison distracts from your own direction. Awareness restores confidence.

Walking your own path does not require certainty or approval. It means trusting that your pace and choices are valid. This trust builds independence.

As you move through the day, notice moments when you feel pulled to measure yourself against others. Allow yourself to return to your own priorities. Confidence strengthens through self-direction.

Personal paths evolve naturally. They respond to lived experience. Self-trust deepens through ownership.

MAY 29

Rest in Self-Trust

Self-trust allows you to rest without constant vigilance or doubt. Today invites you to notice how trust creates ease internally. Rest supports confidence.

Resting in self-trust means allowing yourself to pause without questioning your worth or direction. It allows reassurance to come from within. This steadiness restores energy.

As you move through the day, notice moments when you feel settled in your choices. Allow yourself to rest in that feeling. Confidence deepens through calm.

Self-trust provides stability. It supports restoration. Confidence becomes quieter.

MAY 30

Trust Your Timing

Timing unfolds differently for everyone, shaped by circumstance and readiness. Today invites you to notice whether impatience is overshadowing trust in your process. Awareness restores balance.

Trusting your timing does not mean resisting effort or growth. It means recognizing when readiness aligns naturally. This understanding supports confidence.

As you move through the day, notice moments when waiting feels supportive rather than limiting. Allow yourself to respect your pace. Confidence grows through patience.

Timing aligns through awareness. It cannot be forced. Self-trust deepens with acceptance.

MAY 31

Choose Inner Authority

Inner authority develops when you trust your judgment and values to guide decisions. Today invites you to notice where external influence competes with your own sense of direction. Awareness restores confidence.

Choosing inner authority does not require rejecting advice or collaboration. It means allowing your voice to carry equal weight. This balance strengthens autonomy.

As you move through the day, notice moments when you defer unnecessarily. Allow yourself to claim your perspective. Confidence grows through self-authorization.

Inner authority creates clarity. It reinforces self-trust. The month closes with strength.

JUNE

Balance & Boundaries

June invites a steady recalibration, encouraging you to notice where your energy flows and where it quietly drains. This month focuses on balance that protects well-being and boundaries that support sustainability rather than separation. Care becomes clearer when limits are honored.

Balance is not about perfection or equal distribution, but about responsiveness to your changing needs. Boundaries offer structure that allows energy to be restored and preserved. Together, they create steadiness.

As you move through June, allow balance to feel supportive rather than restrictive. Let boundaries be acts of care rather than defense. Grounding begins with awareness.

JUNE 1

Notice Energy Drains

Energy can be depleted in subtle ways that go unnoticed when days feel full or demanding. Today invites you to observe where your energy feels diminished rather than restored. Awareness is the first step toward balance.

Noticing energy drains does not require immediate correction or judgment. It means paying attention to activities, interactions, or thoughts that consistently leave you feeling tired. This awareness supports clarity.

As you move through the day, notice moments when your energy drops unexpectedly. Allow yourself to acknowledge those patterns without blame. Balance begins with recognition.

Energy awareness supports wiser choices. It reveals where care is needed. Balance grows through noticing.

JUNE 2

Set One Healthy Boundary

Boundaries help protect energy, time, and emotional well-being. Today invites you to consider one boundary that would support balance in your life. Small boundaries create meaningful change.

Setting a healthy boundary does not require confrontation or explanation. It simply means deciding what you can reasonably offer and what you cannot. This clarity supports sustainability.

As you move through the day, notice moments when a boundary feels necessary. Allow yourself to honor it kindly. Boundaries strengthen balance.

Healthy boundaries support self-respect. They reduce strain. Balance becomes possible.

JUNE 3

Balance Giving and Receiving

Giving and receiving are most sustainable when they remain in balance. Today invites you to notice whether your energy is flowing in both directions. Awareness restores equilibrium.

Balancing giving and receiving does not mean withholding care or support. It means allowing yourself to receive help, rest, or acknowledgment without guilt. This openness restores energy.

As you move through the day, notice moments when you give automatically. Allow yourself to receive when it feels appropriate. Balance strengthens through reciprocity.

Balanced exchange supports well-being. It prevents depletion. Care becomes mutual.

JUNE 4

Protect Your Time

Time is a finite resource that shapes how energy is spent or preserved. Today invites you to notice how your time is being used and whether it reflects your priorities. Awareness guides protection.

Protecting your time does not require rigid schedules or withdrawal. It means choosing where your attention goes with intention. This choice supports balance.

As you move through the day, notice moments when your time feels pulled in too many directions. Allow yourself to simplify where possible. Time protection restores clarity.

Respecting time supports energy. It creates space. Balance feels steadier.

JUNE 5

Choose Rest Freely

Rest is often delayed until exhaustion appears. Today invites you to choose rest before depletion occurs. Permission restores balance.

Choosing rest freely means allowing yourself to pause without earning it. It honors your need for recovery as valid and necessary. This choice preserves energy.

As you move through the day, notice when rest feels supportive. Allow yourself to take it without justification. Rest strengthens balance.

Freely chosen rest restores clarity. It supports resilience. Balance becomes sustainable.

JUNE 6

Honor Personal Capacity

Personal capacity changes depending on circumstances, energy, and emotional load. Today invites you to notice what you can realistically offer without strain. Awareness supports balance.

Honoring personal capacity does not mean limitation or failure. It means recognizing your current ability and responding with honesty rather than pressure. This respect preserves energy.

As you move through the day, notice when something feels beyond your capacity. Allow yourself to adjust without guilt. Balance grows through self-honesty.

Respecting capacity prevents burnout. It supports sustainability. Balance becomes kinder.

JUNE 7

Say No Kindly

Saying no can be an act of care rather than rejection. Today invites you to notice where a gentle no protects your energy and time. Kindness strengthens boundaries.

Saying no kindly does not require lengthy explanations or defensiveness. It means responding with clarity while remaining respectful. This approach maintains balance.

As you move through the day, notice moments when saying no feels supportive. Allow yourself to respond calmly and clearly. Boundaries grow stronger through practice.

Kind refusals preserve energy. They protect well-being. Balance remains intact.

JUNE 8

Create Space to Recharge

Recharge happens when space is intentionally created rather than squeezed into exhaustion. Today invites you to notice where space could restore balance. Openness supports renewal.

Creating space to recharge does not require long breaks or major changes. It begins with brief pauses that allow energy to settle. Small spaces matter.

As you move through the day, notice moments when stepping back feels supportive. Allow yourself to take that space without justification. Energy responds to permission.

Space supports restoration. It calms the nervous system. Balance becomes accessible.

JUNE 9

Balance Effort With Ease

Effort becomes sustainable when balanced with ease. Today invites you to notice whether your day allows room for both engagement and rest. Awareness restores equilibrium.

Balancing effort with ease does not mean avoiding responsibility. It means pacing yourself in a way that preserves energy. This balance prevents strain.

As you move through the day, notice moments when easing effort feels supportive. Allow yourself to soften without guilt. Balance grows through flexibility.

Ease enhances effectiveness. It prevents exhaustion. Balance supports continuity.

JUNE 10

Observe Overcommitment

Overcommitment often develops gradually, making it difficult to recognize until exhaustion appears. Today invites you to observe where you may be giving more than feels sustainable. Awareness creates choice.

Observing overcommitment does not require immediate correction. It means noticing patterns of obligation that exceed your capacity. This awareness supports balance.

As you move through the day, notice moments when commitment feels heavy or draining. Allow yourself to acknowledge that experience honestly. Balance begins with observation.

Recognizing overcommitment prevents burnout. It restores clarity. Balance becomes intentional.

JUNE 11

Prioritize Nourishment

Nourishment supports balance when it is treated as a consistent need rather than an occasional reward. Today invites you to notice how well your body and mind are being sustained throughout the day. Awareness restores equilibrium.

Prioritizing nourishment does not mean perfection or strict routines. It means choosing what replenishes you physically, mentally, and emotionally. This attention preserves energy.

As you move through the day, notice how nourishment affects your clarity and stamina. Allow yourself to respond with care rather than delay. Balance strengthens through consistent nourishment.

Nourishment stabilizes energy. It supports resilience. Balance becomes easier to maintain.

JUNE 12

Pause Before Agreeing

Agreements made without pause can quietly strain time and energy. Today invites you to notice the space between request and response. Awareness creates choice.

Pausing before agreeing allows you to check in with capacity, priorities, and intention. It prevents overcommitment without requiring refusal. This pause supports balance.

As you move through the day, notice moments when a pause feels necessary. Allow yourself to take it before responding. Boundaries strengthen through reflection.

Pauses protect energy. They preserve clarity. Balance grows through intention.

JUNE 13

Respect Your Limits

Limits provide structure that supports sustainability rather than restriction. Today invites you to notice where honoring limits preserves your well-being. Respect builds balance.

Respecting limits does not mean avoidance or withdrawal. It means acknowledging what you can offer without compromising yourself. This honesty strengthens boundaries.

As you move through the day, notice moments when limits feel clear. Allow yourself to honor them without apology. Balance responds to self-respect.

Limits protect energy. They support steadiness. Balance becomes grounded.

JUNE 14

Restore Balance Gently

Balance often returns through gentle adjustment rather than forceful change. Today invites you to notice where softness might restore stability. Ease supports renewal.

Restoring balance gently means choosing small corrections instead of drastic measures. It allows energy to settle without disruption. This approach sustains well-being.

As you move through the day, notice moments when gentleness feels supportive. Allow yourself to adjust with care. Balance grows through kindness.

Gentle restoration prevents strain. It honors capacity. Balance becomes sustainable.

JUNE 15

Release Rest Guilt

Rest guilt can undermine recovery and balance. Today invites you to notice beliefs that make rest feel undeserved. Awareness restores permission.

Releasing rest guilt does not mean ignoring responsibility. It means recognizing rest as necessary rather than optional. This shift supports sustainability.

As you move through the day, notice moments when guilt appears around rest. Allow yourself to choose rest anyway. Balance strengthens through permission.

Rest supports clarity. It restores energy. Balance deepens through acceptance.

JUNE 16

Practice Sustainable Living

Sustainability in daily life supports balance when choices consider long-term well-being rather than short-term pressure. Today invites you to notice how your habits affect your energy over time. Awareness encourages steadiness.

Practicing sustainable living does not require drastic change or rigid rules. It means choosing rhythms, commitments, and habits that you can maintain without exhaustion. This approach preserves balance.

As you move through the day, notice where sustainability feels possible. Allow yourself to choose what supports continuity rather than urgency. Balance grows through consistency.

Sustainable choices protect energy. They prevent depletion. Balance becomes enduring.

JUNE 17

Reclaim Personal Time

Personal time allows energy to recover and clarity to return. Today invites you to notice whether you are allowing yourself space that belongs only to you. Awareness restores balance.

Reclaiming personal time does not require withdrawal from responsibility. It means intentionally setting aside moments that are not claimed by obligation. This choice preserves well-being.

As you move through the day, notice where personal time feels necessary. Allow yourself to protect it without explanation. Balance responds to self-respect.

Personal time supports renewal. It restores focus. Balance becomes steadier.

JUNE 18

Choose Balance Today

Balance is shaped by daily choices rather than occasional correction. Today invites you to notice where one small adjustment could restore equilibrium. Awareness creates opportunity.

Choosing balance today does not require perfect conditions. It means responding thoughtfully to what is present right now. This choice supports steadiness.

As you move through the day, notice moments when imbalance feels apparent. Allow yourself to respond gently. Balance grows through responsiveness.

Daily balance builds resilience. It supports well-being. Balance becomes practiced.

JUNE 19

Trust Boundaries as Care

Boundaries are expressions of care rather than distance. Today invites you to notice how boundaries protect energy and relationships. Awareness reframes limits.

Trusting boundaries as care does not mean rejecting connection. It means creating structure that allows engagement to remain healthy. This perspective supports balance.

As you move through the day, notice moments when boundaries feel supportive. Allow yourself to trust their role. Balance strengthens through clarity.

Boundaries preserve energy. They support respect. Balance becomes relational.

JUNE 20

Reduce Daily Overload

Daily overload can accumulate quietly until balance feels difficult to restore. Today invites you to notice where demands exceed capacity. Awareness creates relief.

Reducing daily overload does not require eliminating all responsibility. It means identifying areas where simplification is possible. This choice restores balance.

As you move through the day, notice moments when tasks feel overwhelming. Allow yourself to reduce or delay where possible. Balance responds to moderation.

Reduced overload supports clarity. It protects energy. Balance becomes achievable.

JUNE 21

Practice Energy Awareness

Energy awareness begins with noticing how your body and mind respond throughout the day. Today invites you to observe shifts in energy without trying to correct them immediately. Awareness creates balance.

Practicing energy awareness does not require constant monitoring. It means gently checking in with yourself at different moments. This attention supports wiser choices.

As you move through the day, notice when your energy rises or falls. Allow that information to guide your pace and expectations. Balance grows through attentiveness.

Energy awareness supports sustainability. It prevents unnecessary strain. Balance becomes intuitive.

JUNE 22

Allow Space to Breathe

Breathing space is essential for balance, even when days feel full. Today invites you to notice where you can create small pauses. Space restores clarity.

Allowing space to breathe does not require long breaks. It means permitting moments of stillness or quiet between activities. These pauses support equilibrium.

As you move through the day, notice moments when tension builds. Allow yourself to pause and breathe. Balance responds to space.

Breathing space calms the nervous system. It restores presence. Balance becomes steadier.

JUNE 23

Simplify Obligations

Obligations can multiply until they quietly overwhelm capacity. Today invites you to notice which commitments truly require your attention. Simplification restores balance.

Simplifying obligations does not mean neglecting responsibility. It means choosing where your energy is most effectively used. This choice supports sustainability.

As you move through the day, notice obligations that feel heavy or unnecessary. Allow yourself to adjust where possible. Balance responds to clarity.

Simplified commitments protect energy. They reduce overwhelm. Balance becomes manageable.

JUNE 24

Protect Emotional Space

Emotional space allows you to respond thoughtfully rather than reactively. Today invites you to notice where emotional boundaries support well-being. Protection preserves balance.

Protecting emotional space does not mean avoiding connection. It means choosing how much emotional energy you extend in certain situations. This discernment supports resilience.

As you move through the day, notice moments when emotional space feels compromised. Allow yourself to step back gently. Balance strengthens through protection.

Emotional space supports clarity. It prevents exhaustion. Balance becomes sustainable.

JUNE 25

End the Month Grounded

As the month moves toward its close, today invites you to notice how balance and boundaries have supported you. Reflection allows grounding to settle. Awareness replaces urgency.

Ending the month grounded does not require evaluation or judgment. It means acknowledging steadiness where it exists. Recognition strengthens integration.

As you move through the day, notice moments when you feel more centered than before. Allow yourself to honor that feeling. Grounding deepens through acknowledgment.

Grounded endings support continuity. They prepare you to move forward. Balance feels integrated.

JUNE 26

Carry Balance Forward

Balance becomes most meaningful when it continues beyond a single moment or month. Today invites you to notice which practices and boundaries you want to carry forward. Continuity supports stability.

Carrying balance forward does not mean maintaining rigid control. It means staying attentive to what supports well-being as circumstances change. This flexibility preserves energy.

As you move through the day, notice habits that feel worth sustaining. Allow yourself to commit gently rather than forcefully. Balance strengthens through consistency.

Sustained balance feels adaptable. It evolves with your needs. Well-being remains supported.

JUNE 27

Respect Your Pace

Your pace reflects capacity, energy, and circumstance rather than weakness or delay. Today invites you to notice whether you are honoring your natural rhythm. Respect restores balance.

Respecting your pace does not mean resisting growth. It means allowing progress to unfold without pressure or comparison. This approach supports sustainability.

As you move through the day, notice moments when slowing down feels supportive. Allow yourself to adjust without guilt. Balance responds to self-respect.

A respected pace prevents exhaustion. It supports clarity. Balance becomes humane.

JUNE 28

Choose Alignment Over Pressure

Pressure can distort priorities and drain energy. Today invites you to notice where alignment offers a steadier guide than urgency. Awareness restores balance.

Choosing alignment over pressure means acting in ways that reflect values rather than demands. It allows decisions to feel grounded rather than reactive. This clarity supports well-being.

As you move through the day, notice moments when pressure arises. Allow yourself to pause and choose alignment instead. Balance grows through intention.

Alignment reduces strain. It preserves energy. Balance feels authentic.

JUNE 29

Rest Before Burnout

Burnout often appears after prolonged neglect of rest. Today invites you to choose rest proactively rather than reactively. Prevention supports balance.

Resting before burnout does not mean avoiding responsibility. It means recognizing early signs of fatigue and responding with care. This awareness preserves energy.

As you move through the day, notice when rest would be supportive. Allow yourself to take it without waiting for exhaustion. Balance strengthens through foresight.

Proactive rest protects resilience. It sustains capacity. Balance becomes preventive.

JUNE 30

Maintain Healthy Distance

Healthy distance allows relationships and responsibilities to remain sustainable. Today invites you to notice where space supports clarity and respect. Distance can be caring.

Maintaining healthy distance does not mean disengagement or withdrawal. It means choosing appropriate closeness that preserves emotional well-being. This discernment supports balance.

As you move through the day, notice moments when stepping back feels supportive. Allow yourself to create space gently. Balance responds to discernment.

Healthy distance protects energy. It supports clarity and respect. The month closes grounded and steady.

JULY

Presence & Joy

July invites you to soften your attention and return to the present moment, where joy often exists quietly without needing to be created or pursued. This month focuses on experiencing life as it unfolds, allowing presence to replace pressure and enjoyment to feel natural. Joy here is gentle, accessible, and rooted in awareness.

Presence does not require constant effort or discipline. It emerges when you stop rushing past your own experience. Joy becomes easier when you allow yourself to notice it.

As you move through July, let presence guide your pace. Allow joy to appear without expectation. Being here is enough.

JULY 1

Be Fully Here

Being fully here means allowing your attention to settle into the present moment rather than drifting toward what has passed or what might come next. Today invites you to notice where your awareness rests throughout the day. Presence creates openness.

Being fully here does not require effort or concentration. It means gently returning your attention to what you are experiencing right now. This return supports calm and clarity.

As you move through the day, notice moments when your mind wanders away from the present. Allow yourself to come back without judgment. Presence deepens through repetition.

Being here anchors experience. It reduces strain. Joy often appears naturally.

JULY 2

Notice Simple Pleasures

Simple pleasures often pass unnoticed when attention is elsewhere. Today invites you to slow down enough to notice small moments that bring comfort or ease. Awareness restores appreciation.

Noticing simple pleasures does not require seeking them out. It means recognizing what is already present. This recognition supports contentment.

As you move through the day, notice sensory experiences that feel pleasant or grounding. Allow yourself to linger briefly. Joy grows through attention.

Simple pleasures soften experience. They invite calm. Presence enhances enjoyment.

JULY 3

Let Joy Be Easy

Joy does not need to be earned or intensified to be meaningful. Today invites you to allow joy to arise without effort or expectation. Ease supports happiness.

Letting joy be easy means releasing the belief that joy must be dramatic or constant. It allows moments of lightness to be enough. This permission reduces pressure.

As you move through the day, notice when something brings a subtle sense of enjoyment. Allow yourself to accept it without questioning. Joy responds to openness.

Ease allows joy to settle. It feels natural and steady. Presence supports happiness.

JULY 4

Savor One Moment

Moments pass quickly when attention is divided. Today invites you to savor one moment fully, allowing it to unfold without interruption. Focus deepens experience.

Savoring does not require prolonging or capturing the moment. It means being attentive while it is happening. This presence enhances meaning.

As you move through the day, notice a moment that feels worth savoring. Allow yourself to remain present until it naturally ends. Joy strengthens through focus.

Savoring slows time internally. It deepens awareness. Presence enriches joy.

JULY 5

Laugh Freely

Laughter can restore lightness and release tension without explanation. Today invites you to allow laughter when it arises naturally. Joy responds to openness.

Laughing freely does not require humor to be forced or shared. It means allowing amusement or delight to express itself. This freedom supports ease.

As you move through the day, notice moments that invite laughter or smiling. Allow yourself to respond without restraint. Lightness replenishes energy.

Laughter relaxes the body. It clears emotional weight. Joy feels more accessible.

JULY 6

Practice Light Gratitude

Gratitude can feel heavy when it becomes another obligation rather than a quiet noticing. Today invites you to approach gratitude lightly, without searching for meaning or significance. Ease keeps gratitude sincere.

Practicing light gratitude means acknowledging what feels supportive without turning it into a lesson. It allows appreciation to arise naturally instead of being constructed. This approach preserves joy.

As you move through the day, notice small moments that feel pleasant or supportive. Allow yourself to recognize them briefly. Gratitude grows through gentle awareness.

Light gratitude softens experience. It does not demand reflection. Joy responds to simplicity.

JULY 7

Enjoy Unstructured Time

Unstructured time allows presence to unfold without direction or expectation. Today invites you to notice how it feels to let moments exist without planning or productivity. Freedom restores joy.

Enjoying unstructured time does not mean avoiding responsibility. It means allowing space where nothing needs to be accomplished. This openness supports renewal.

As you move through the day, notice opportunities to be without agenda. Allow yourself to remain there briefly. Presence deepens without effort.

Unstructured time refreshes awareness. It invites ease. Joy often appears quietly.

JULY 8

Welcome Spontaneous Happiness

Happiness sometimes appears unexpectedly, without cause or preparation. Today invites you to welcome those moments instead of questioning or analyzing them. Openness sustains joy.

Welcoming spontaneous happiness means allowing enjoyment to exist without needing justification. It allows lightness to be experienced fully. This acceptance supports presence.

As you move through the day, notice moments of unplanned happiness. Allow yourself to receive them without interruption. Joy strengthens through permission.

Spontaneous happiness feels fleeting yet real. It thrives when noticed. Presence makes room for delight.

JULY 9

Presence Over Productivity

Productivity can pull attention away from lived experience. Today invites you to prioritize presence even while completing tasks. Awareness restores balance.

Choosing presence over productivity does not mean neglecting responsibility. It means staying connected to yourself while doing what needs to be done. This connection supports well-being.

As you move through the day, notice moments when speed replaces awareness. Allow yourself to slow slightly and return to the present. Joy often emerges through presence.

Presence enriches action. It reduces strain. Joy becomes more accessible.

JULY 10

Breathe Summer Ease

Breath reflects the pace at which you are living. Today invites you to breathe in a way that matches the ease of summer rather than urgency or tension. Breath restores calm.

Breathing summer ease means allowing inhalations and exhalations to feel unforced. It invites relaxation without instruction. This softness supports joy.

As you move through the day, notice moments when your breath becomes shallow or hurried. Allow it to slow gently. Ease spreads through awareness.

Ease begins with breath. It calms the body. Joy feels more available.

JULY 11

Let Playfulness Lead

Playfulness brings a sense of lightness that can soften even ordinary moments. Today invites you to allow curiosity and ease to guide how you engage with your day. Letting playfulness lead restores balance.

Letting playfulness lead does not mean avoiding responsibility or structure. It means approaching tasks and interactions with flexibility rather than rigidity. This shift supports joy.

As you move through the day, notice moments when playfulness feels possible. Allow yourself to respond with openness rather than restraint. Joy grows through permission.

Playfulness refreshes perspective. It loosens pressure. Presence becomes more enjoyable.

JULY 12

Appreciate Everyday Beauty

Beauty often exists quietly within ordinary surroundings. Today invites you to notice colors, textures, sounds, or moments that are easy to overlook. Attention restores appreciation.

Appreciating everyday beauty does not require seeking special experiences. It means noticing what is already present. This awareness deepens joy.

As you move through the day, notice small details that feel pleasing or grounding. Allow yourself to acknowledge them without rushing past. Presence enhances enjoyment.

Everyday beauty softens experience. It brings calm. Joy becomes more accessible.

JULY 13

Experience Without Rushing

Rushing can disconnect you from what you are actually experiencing. Today invites you to slow down enough to fully inhabit moments as they unfold. Presence deepens awareness.

Experiencing without rushing does not require dramatic slowing or withdrawal. It means giving yourself permission to be where you are. This allowance supports joy.

As you move through the day, notice moments when you hurry unnecessarily. Allow yourself to ease your pace when possible. Joy responds to steadiness.

Slower experiences feel richer. They allow meaning to surface. Presence strengthens joy.

JULY 14

Reconnect With Wonder

Wonder often fades when familiarity takes over attention. Today invites you to look again with curiosity rather than assumption. Freshness restores joy.

Reconnecting with wonder does not require novelty or travel. It means allowing yourself to be surprised by what is already around you. This openness supports presence.

As you move through the day, notice moments when curiosity arises naturally. Allow yourself to linger there. Joy grows through wonder.

Wonder refreshes perception. It softens routine. Presence becomes lighter.

JULY 15

Celebrate Being Alive

Being alive is experienced through sensation, movement, and awareness. Today invites you to notice the simple fact of existence without needing justification. Awareness deepens gratitude.

Celebrating being alive does not require dramatic emotion. It means acknowledging breath, sensation, and presence. This recognition supports joy.

As you move through the day, notice moments when aliveness feels clear. Allow yourself to acknowledge them gently. Joy responds to awareness.

Life is felt moment by moment. Presence makes it vivid. Joy grows quietly.

JULY 16

Let Joy Be Quiet

Joy does not always need expression or excitement to be real. Today invites you to notice quiet moments of ease that exist without announcement. Stillness allows joy to settle.

Letting joy be quiet means allowing contentment to exist without explaining or amplifying it. It honors subtle satisfaction rather than seeking intensity. This gentleness supports presence.

As you move through the day, notice moments when calm feels pleasant. Allow yourself to remain there without distraction. Joy deepens through stillness.

Quiet joy feels steady. It does not demand attention. Presence makes space for it.

JULY 17

Notice Contentment Now

Contentment often exists before you think to look for it. Today invites you to notice whether satisfaction is already present in small, ordinary ways. Awareness restores appreciation.

Noticing contentment does not mean denying difficulty or challenge. It means allowing space for what feels sufficient in this moment. This balance supports joy.

As you move through the day, notice moments when nothing feels missing. Allow yourself to acknowledge that feeling. Joy grows through recognition.

Contentment softens desire. It steadies attention. Presence supports ease.

JULY 18

Stay Curious Today

Curiosity keeps experience open and flexible. Today invites you to approach familiar moments with interest rather than assumption. Curiosity refreshes presence.

Staying curious does not require constant questioning. It means allowing yourself to notice without immediately labeling or concluding. This openness supports joy.

As you move through the day, notice moments when curiosity feels natural. Allow yourself to follow it briefly. Joy responds to engagement.

Curiosity renews attention. It keeps experience light. Presence feels alive.

JULY 19

Enjoy the Ordinary

Ordinary moments often hold quiet pleasure when attention is available. Today invites you to notice how routine experiences can feel satisfying without needing change. Presence restores enjoyment.

Enjoying the ordinary does not require reframing or effort. It means allowing yourself to fully experience what is already happening. This simplicity supports joy.

As you move through the day, notice moments that feel comfortably familiar. Allow yourself to appreciate them without rushing past. Joy grows through acceptance.

The ordinary carries comfort. It grounds experience. Presence deepens enjoyment.

JULY 20

Smile Without Reason

Smiling can arise naturally without cause or explanation. Today invites you to allow that expression when it appears. Ease supports joy.

Smiling without reason does not require happiness to be justified. It means allowing lightness to pass through without analysis. This permission softens experience.

As you move through the day, notice moments when a smile appears spontaneously. Allow yourself to follow it gently. Joy spreads through openness.

Smiles relax the body. They invite warmth. Presence amplifies lightness.

JULY 21

Choose Joy Gently

Joy often arrives more naturally when it is invited rather than pursued. Today invites you to approach joy with gentleness, allowing it to appear in its own time. Softness supports presence.

Choosing joy gently does not mean ignoring difficulty or forcing positivity. It means remaining open to moments of ease without demanding that they last. This openness sustains joy.

As you move through the day, notice where joy feels possible without effort. Allow yourself to welcome it lightly. Joy responds to gentleness.

Gentle joy feels steady. It does not exhaust attention. Presence keeps it accessible.

JULY 22

Create Light Moments

Light moments can soften the texture of a day without changing its structure. Today invites you to notice where small shifts can bring ease or relief. Awareness creates lightness.

Creating light moments does not require special circumstances. It means allowing humor, softness, or ease to enter ordinary situations. This choice supports joy.

As you move through the day, notice opportunities to lighten your experience. Allow yourself to take them without hesitation. Joy grows through simplicity.

Light moments refresh perspective. They reduce heaviness. Presence supports ease.

JULY 23

Stay Present Always

Presence anchors experience even when circumstances shift. Today invites you to return to the present moment repeatedly throughout the day. Attention steadies awareness.

Staying present does not mean constant focus or control. It means gently noticing when attention drifts and returning without judgment. This practice supports joy.

As you move through the day, notice moments when you reconnect with now. Allow yourself to remain briefly. Presence deepens contentment.

Presence grounds experience. It reduces strain. Joy becomes more available.

JULY 24

End the Month Joyful

As the month begins to close, today invites you to notice how joy has shown up in quiet and unexpected ways. Reflection allows enjoyment to settle. Awareness replaces urgency.

Ending the month joyful does not require constant happiness. It means acknowledging moments of lightness and presence that have occurred. Recognition strengthens joy.

As you move through the day, notice what feels lighter than before. Allow yourself to honor that shift. Joy carries forward through acknowledgment.

Joyful endings support continuity. They prepare the way ahead. Presence feels complete.

JULY 25

Carry Joy Forward

Joy becomes more sustainable when it is carried gently rather than held tightly. Today invites you to notice what helps joy remain accessible beyond the moment. Continuity supports ease.

Carrying joy forward does not mean preserving every feeling. It means staying open to joy as circumstances change. This openness supports presence.

As you move through the day, notice habits or attitudes that support joy. Allow yourself to continue them naturally. Joy grows through consistency.

Sustained joy feels flexible. It adapts with experience. Presence keeps it alive.

JULY 26

Let Happiness Be Simple

Happiness often becomes complicated when it is expected to look a certain way. Today invites you to allow happiness to feel uncomplicated and accessible. Simplicity supports presence.

Letting happiness be simple means releasing the need for intensity or explanation. It allows small moments of ease to be enough. This permission supports joy.

As you move through the day, notice moments that feel quietly satisfying. Allow yourself to accept them without adding meaning. Happiness settles through simplicity.

Simple happiness feels steady. It does not demand effort. Presence makes room for it.

JULY 27

Be Where You Are

Attention often drifts toward what is next or what has passed. Today invites you to be fully where you are, without mentally leaving the moment. Presence restores connection.

Being where you are does not require effort or control. It means noticing your surroundings, sensations, and breath as they are. This awareness supports joy.

As you move through the day, notice moments when you return to now. Allow yourself to remain briefly. Presence deepens experience.

Being here grounds awareness. It softens urgency. Joy becomes more available.

JULY 28

Welcome Ease

Ease can feel unfamiliar when effort has become habitual. Today invites you to notice where ease is already present. Awareness restores softness.

Welcoming ease does not mean avoiding responsibility. It means releasing unnecessary tension in how you approach what you are doing. This shift supports joy.

As you move through the day, notice moments when things flow without struggle. Allow yourself to remain there. Ease replenishes energy.

Ease relaxes the body. It calms the mind. Presence supports lightness.

JULY 29

Pause to Enjoy

Enjoyment deepens when you pause long enough to notice it. Today invites you to slow briefly and allow enjoyment to register. Pausing enhances presence.

Pausing to enjoy does not require stopping everything. It means giving attention to what feels pleasant or meaningful. This awareness supports joy.

As you move through the day, notice moments worth pausing for. Allow yourself to linger briefly. Enjoyment grows through attention.

Pauses enrich experience. They anchor awareness. Joy becomes more vivid.

JULY 30

Rest in Presence

Presence can be a place of rest rather than effort. Today invites you to notice how simply being aware can feel restorative. Stillness supports joy.

Resting in presence means allowing yourself to stop striving for improvement or outcome. It allows experience to be enough as it is. This acceptance restores balance.

As you move through the day, notice moments when awareness feels calming. Allow yourself to settle there. Presence replenishes energy.

Presence offers rest. It steadies attention. Joy feels supported.

JULY 31

Close the Month Present

As July comes to a close, today invites you to pause and notice how presence and joy have shaped your experience. Reflection allows awareness to integrate. Ending gently supports continuity.

Closing the month present does not require evaluation or summary. It means acknowledging moments of attention, lightness, and ease. Recognition deepens appreciation.

As you move through the day, notice what feels complete or settled. Allow yourself to honor that feeling. Presence carries forward naturally.

Present endings feel grounded. They prepare what comes next. Joy remains accessible.

AUGUST

Calm & Resilience

August invites a steadier kind of strength, one that remains present even when circumstances feel demanding or uncertain. This month focuses on cultivating calm that does not disappear under pressure and resilience that grows quietly through consistency and care. Stability becomes a practice rather than a reaction.

Calm is not the absence of challenge, but the ability to meet challenge without becoming overwhelmed by it. Resilience develops through awareness, patience, and the willingness to recover gently rather than push relentlessly. Together, they create emotional steadiness.

As you move through August, allow calm to anchor you and resilience to support you. Let steadiness replace urgency. Strength grows quietly through presence.

AUGUST 1

Practice Emotional Steadiness

Emotional steadiness allows you to remain present with your experience without being pulled too far by reaction. Today invites you to notice how your emotions move and settle throughout the day. Awareness supports balance.

Practicing emotional steadiness does not mean suppressing feelings or avoiding intensity. It means allowing emotions to exist without letting them dictate every response. This approach builds resilience.

As you move through the day, notice moments when you feel centered despite change. Allow yourself to acknowledge that steadiness. Calm grows through recognition.

Emotional steadiness supports clarity. It prevents overwhelm. Resilience develops gradually.

AUGUST 2

Stay Grounded Under Pressure

Pressure can make attention scatter and reactions intensify. Today invites you to remain grounded even when demands increase. Grounding supports calm.

Staying grounded under pressure does not mean eliminating stress. It means anchoring yourself in breath, body, and present awareness. This anchoring strengthens resilience.

As you move through the day, notice moments when pressure rises. Allow yourself to return to what feels solid and stable. Calm responds to grounding.

Grounded attention reduces reactivity. It preserves clarity. Resilience strengthens through steadiness.

AUGUST 3

Respond Calmly

Calm responses often emerge when you pause long enough to choose them. Today invites you to notice the space between stimulus and reaction. Awareness creates choice.

Responding calmly does not require perfection or constant control. It means allowing yourself a moment to settle before engaging. This pause supports resilience.

As you move through the day, notice moments when you respond with intention rather than impulse. Allow yourself to recognize that effort. Calm grows through practice.

Calm responses protect energy. They reduce conflict. Resilience becomes consistent.

AUGUST 4

Rest Before Exhaustion

Exhaustion often arrives after long periods of ignoring early signals. Today invites you to rest before depletion becomes unavoidable. Prevention supports resilience.

Resting before exhaustion does not mean avoiding responsibility. It means recognizing limits early and responding with care. This awareness preserves calm.

As you move through the day, notice signs of fatigue before they intensify. Allow yourself to pause or slow down. Calm responds to foresight.

Early rest sustains strength. It prevents burnout. Resilience becomes protective.

AUGUST 5

Trust Coping Skills

You have developed ways to cope through experience and adaptation. Today invites you to trust those skills rather than doubting your ability to manage difficulty. Confidence supports calm.

Trusting coping skills does not mean expecting ease at all times. It means remembering that you have navigated challenges before. This memory builds resilience.

As you move through the day, notice moments when you rely on familiar coping strategies. Allow yourself to acknowledge their effectiveness. Calm grows through trust.

Coping skills strengthen with use. They provide reassurance. Resilience feels accessible.

AUGUST 6

Breathe Through Discomfort

Discomfort can feel overwhelming when it is met with resistance or urgency. Today invites you to stay present with discomfort long enough to notice how breath can support steadiness. Awareness reduces intensity.

Breathing through discomfort does not mean forcing calm or dismissing what you feel. It means allowing the breath to create space around sensation and emotion. This space supports resilience.

As you move through the day, notice moments of discomfort as they arise. Allow your breath to remain slow and supportive. Calm grows through presence.

Breath anchors awareness. It softens reactivity. Resilience strengthens through steadiness.

AUGUST 7

Strengthen Inner Stability

Inner stability provides a sense of grounding that remains available even when circumstances shift. Today invites you to notice where stability already exists within you. Recognition builds calm.

Strengthening inner stability does not require eliminating uncertainty. It means cultivating steadiness through awareness, routine, and self-trust. This steadiness supports resilience.

As you move through the day, notice moments when you feel centered despite external change. Allow yourself to acknowledge that stability. Calm deepens through awareness.

Inner stability offers reliability. It reduces emotional swing. Resilience becomes dependable.

AUGUST 8

Choose Calm Over Control

The desire for control often increases when uncertainty appears. Today invites you to choose calm instead of tightening your grip on outcomes. Calm restores clarity.

Choosing calm over control does not mean disengaging or giving up responsibility. It means releasing unnecessary tension while remaining present. This choice supports resilience.

As you move through the day, notice moments when control feels tempting. Allow yourself to soften and return to calm. Calm responds to release.

Control exhausts energy. Calm preserves it. Resilience grows through trust.

AUGUST 9

Recover Gently

Recovery happens most effectively when it is approached with gentleness rather than urgency. Today invites you to notice how softness supports healing and renewal. Gentleness restores balance.

Recovering gently does not require immediate improvement or resolution. It means allowing time, rest, and patience to do their work. This approach supports resilience.

As you move through the day, notice moments when gentleness feels appropriate. Allow yourself to respond with care rather than pressure. Calm grows through compassion.

Gentle recovery respects capacity. It prevents further strain. Resilience becomes sustainable.

AUGUST 10

Accept What Is

Acceptance can reduce suffering when circumstances feel difficult or unchangeable. Today invites you to notice where resistance increases tension unnecessarily. Acceptance restores calm.

Accepting what is does not mean approving or giving up. It means acknowledging reality as it exists in this moment. This acknowledgment supports resilience.

As you move through the day, notice moments when acceptance feels possible. Allow yourself to release resistance gently. Calm responds to honesty.

Acceptance steadies emotion. It reduces struggle. Resilience strengthens through truth.

AUGUST 11

Build Quiet Resilience

Resilience often develops in subtle ways that are easy to overlook. Today invites you to notice how you continue showing up, adapting, and steadying yourself through ordinary challenges. Awareness strengthens calm.

Building quiet resilience does not require dramatic effort or visible struggle. It grows through patience, consistency, and self-support over time. This process supports emotional steadiness.

As you move through the day, notice moments when you recover more quickly than before. Allow yourself to recognize that progress. Calm deepens through acknowledgment.

Quiet resilience feels reliable. It does not seek attention. Strength grows steadily.

AUGUST 12

Stay Present in Challenge

Challenges can pull attention toward fear or future outcomes. Today invites you to remain present with what is happening now rather than imagining what may come next. Presence steadies emotion.

Staying present in challenge does not mean denying difficulty. It means anchoring yourself in breath, body, and awareness. This grounding supports resilience.

As you move through the day, notice moments when attention drifts into worry. Allow yourself to return to the present gently. Calm responds to presence.

Presence reduces overwhelm. It supports clarity. Resilience strengthens through attention.

AUGUST 13

Balance Strength and Softness

Strength and softness can exist together without conflict. Today invites you to notice where firmness and gentleness can support each other. Balance restores calm.

Balancing strength and softness does not require choosing one over the other. It means responding flexibly based on what the moment needs. This adaptability supports resilience.

As you move through the day, notice moments when softness enhances strength. Allow yourself to trust that balance. Calm grows through integration.

Balanced responses feel humane. They prevent rigidity. Resilience becomes adaptable.

AUGUST 14

Restore Emotional Energy

Emotional energy can be depleted through prolonged stress or intensity. Today invites you to notice what restores your emotional reserves. Awareness supports recovery.

Restoring emotional energy does not require solving problems or fixing situations. It means allowing space for rest, expression, or comfort. This care supports resilience.

As you move through the day, notice moments when emotional relief feels possible. Allow yourself to receive it without guilt. Calm responds to replenishment.

Emotional restoration supports stability. It prevents burnout. Resilience becomes sustainable.

AUGUST 15

Practice Inner Calm

Inner calm is a skill that develops through repeated attention rather than force. Today invites you to notice how calm feels in your body and mind. Awareness builds steadiness.

Practicing inner calm does not require eliminating emotion or challenge. It means creating moments of stillness within movement. This practice supports resilience.

As you move through the day, notice moments when calm feels accessible. Allow yourself to return there briefly. Calm strengthens through familiarity.

Inner calm steadies response. It supports clarity. Resilience grows quietly.

AUGUST 16

Trust Your Recovery

Recovery often unfolds gradually rather than all at once. Today invites you to notice how your ability to recover has strengthened through experience and care. Trust supports calm.

Trusting your recovery does not mean expecting immediate relief or resolution. It means believing in your capacity to return to balance over time. This belief supports resilience.

As you move through the day, notice moments when you regain steadiness after difficulty. Allow yourself to acknowledge that recovery. Calm grows through trust.

Recovery reinforces confidence. It restores balance. Resilience deepens through experience.

AUGUST 17

Pause When Needed

Pausing creates space for awareness and choice. Today invites you to notice when a pause would support steadiness rather than delay. Awareness restores calm.

Pausing when needed does not mean stopping progress or avoiding responsibility. It means allowing space for regulation and clarity. This pause supports resilience.

As you move through the day, notice moments when tension builds. Allow yourself to pause before continuing. Calm responds to permission.

Pauses protect energy. They support clarity. Resilience becomes sustainable.

AUGUST 18

Stay Patient With Stress

Stress can challenge patience when it lingers or intensifies. Today invites you to meet stress with patience rather than urgency. Patience steadies emotion.

Staying patient with stress does not mean tolerating harm or ignoring needs. It means allowing your nervous system time to settle. This patience supports resilience.

As you move through the day, notice moments when stress feels persistent. Allow yourself to respond slowly and thoughtfully. Calm grows through patience.

Patience reduces escalation. It preserves energy. Resilience strengthens quietly.

AUGUST 19

Allow Emotional Space

Emotional space allows feelings to move without becoming overwhelming. Today invites you to notice where space would support steadiness. Openness restores calm.

Allowing emotional space does not mean disengaging or suppressing emotion. It means permitting feelings to exist without immediate action. This allowance supports resilience.

As you move through the day, notice moments when emotions feel crowded. Allow yourself to create space gently. Calm responds to openness.

Emotional space supports clarity. It prevents overload. Resilience becomes accessible.

AUGUST 20

Recenter After Difficulty

Difficulty can temporarily pull you away from balance. Today invites you to notice how you return to center after challenge. Awareness restores calm.

Recentering after difficulty does not require immediate resolution. It means allowing yourself to settle back into steadiness gradually. This process supports resilience.

As you move through the day, notice moments when equilibrium returns. Allow yourself to acknowledge that shift. Calm grows through recognition.

Recentering restores orientation. It supports stability. Resilience strengthens over time.

AUGUST 21

End the Month Steady

As the month begins to move toward its close, today invites you to notice how steadiness has supported you through change and challenge. Reflection allows calm to settle more deeply. Awareness replaces urgency.

Ending the month steady does not require everything to feel resolved or complete. It means recognizing moments where you remained grounded despite difficulty. This recognition strengthens resilience.

As you move through the day, notice where steadiness feels more accessible than before. Allow yourself to acknowledge that shift. Calm deepens through recognition.

Steady endings create integration. They support continuity. Resilience feels embodied.

AUGUST 22

Carry Resilience Forward

Resilience becomes most supportive when it continues beyond a single moment or situation. Today invites you to notice which practices help you recover and remain steady. Continuity strengthens calm.

Carrying resilience forward does not mean staying guarded or tense. It means trusting your ability to adapt and respond with care. This trust supports balance.

As you move through the day, notice habits that support recovery and steadiness. Allow yourself to continue them gently. Calm grows through consistency.

Resilience carried forward feels flexible. It adapts to circumstance. Strength remains available.

AUGUST 23

Breathe Before Reacting

Reactivity often arises when breath becomes shallow or hurried. Today invites you to pause and breathe before responding. Breath creates space.

Breathing before reacting does not require control or suppression. It means allowing one full breath to settle the nervous system. This pause supports resilience.

As you move through the day, notice moments when emotion rises quickly. Allow yourself to breathe before speaking or acting. Calm responds to breath.

Breath steadies response. It reduces escalation. Resilience strengthens through pause.

AUGUST 24

Trust Yourself Under Pressure

Pressure can cause self-doubt even when experience supports you. Today invites you to trust your ability to navigate demanding moments. Confidence restores calm.

Trusting yourself under pressure does not mean expecting flawless outcomes. It means remembering that you have adapted before. This remembrance supports resilience.

As you move through the day, notice moments when pressure increases. Allow yourself to rely on your judgment. Calm grows through trust.

Self-trust anchors response. It steadies emotion. Resilience becomes reliable.

AUGUST 25

Calm Is a Choice

Calm can feel elusive when circumstances feel intense. Today invites you to notice where calm remains available as a choice rather than a condition. Awareness restores agency.

Recognizing calm as a choice does not mean ignoring emotion or difficulty. It means choosing how you relate to what arises. This perspective supports resilience.

As you move through the day, notice moments when you consciously choose calm. Allow yourself to acknowledge that choice. Calm strengthens through intention.

Chosen calm feels empowering. It restores balance. Resilience becomes practiced.

AUGUST 26

Return to Stillness

Stillness offers a place where the nervous system can reset and settle. Today invites you to return to moments of quiet without needing to fix or resolve anything. Stillness restores calm.

Returning to stillness does not require silence or withdrawal from life. It means allowing brief pauses where nothing is demanded of you. This allowance supports resilience.

As you move through the day, notice moments when stillness feels accessible. Allow yourself to remain there briefly. Calm grows through quiet presence.

Stillness stabilizes emotion. It supports clarity. Resilience deepens gently.

AUGUST 27

Maintain Inner Balance

Inner balance helps you move through change without losing your center. Today invites you to notice how balance feels internally rather than externally. Awareness restores steadiness.

Maintaining inner balance does not mean keeping emotions neutral or flat. It means allowing feelings to move while staying anchored within yourself. This anchoring supports resilience.

As you move through the day, notice moments when balance feels intact. Allow yourself to recognize that steadiness. Calm strengthens through acknowledgment.

Inner balance supports regulation. It reduces overwhelm. Resilience remains available.

AUGUST 28

Choose Calm Consistently

Calm becomes more accessible when it is chosen repeatedly rather than occasionally. Today invites you to notice how consistency supports emotional steadiness. Repetition strengthens resilience.

Choosing calm consistently does not mean suppressing reactions. It means returning to calm again and again when disruption occurs. This return builds stability.

As you move through the day, notice moments when calm is restored after disturbance. Allow yourself to acknowledge that effort. Calm grows through practice.

Consistent calm builds trust. It steadies response. Resilience becomes dependable.

AUGUST 29

Honor Emotional Recovery

Emotional recovery deserves recognition just as much as effort or endurance. Today invites you to notice how recovery unfolds within you. Awareness restores balance.

Honoring emotional recovery does not mean expecting linear progress. It means allowing space for fluctuation and rest. This compassion supports resilience.

As you move through the day, notice moments when emotions feel lighter or more settled. Allow yourself to recognize that shift. Calm responds to care.

Recovery renews capacity. It supports clarity. Resilience grows with patience.

AUGUST 30

Let Steadiness Lead

Steadiness offers guidance when situations feel uncertain or demanding. Today invites you to allow steadiness rather than urgency to guide your responses. Calm restores orientation.

Letting steadiness lead does not mean avoiding action. It means responding at a pace that preserves balance. This approach supports resilience.

As you move through the day, notice moments when steadiness influences your choices. Allow yourself to trust that guidance. Calm deepens through alignment.

Steady leadership reduces strain. It supports clarity. Resilience remains grounded.

AUGUST 31

Close the Month Calm

As August comes to a close, today invites you to reflect on how calm and resilience have supported you. Reflection allows steadiness to integrate fully. Ending gently supports continuity.

Closing the month calm does not require evaluation or conclusion. It means acknowledging moments of balance, recovery, and presence. Recognition strengthens calm.

As you move through the day, notice what feels settled or steadier than before. Allow yourself to honor that progress. Calm carries forward naturally.

Calm endings feel grounded. They prepare the next phase. Resilience remains within reach.

SEPTEMBER

Reflection & Focus

September invites a natural turning inward, offering space to reflect on what has unfolded and to clarify where attention is best directed next. This month emphasizes thoughtful focus that grows from awareness rather than urgency. Reflection becomes a source of guidance.

Focus here is not about narrowing life, but about aligning energy with what feels meaningful and sustaining. Reflection allows insight to emerge without pressure or judgment. Together, they support clarity.

As you move through September, allow yourself to pause, review, and refine gently. Let focus feel intentional rather than forced. Insight grows through attention.

SEPTEMBER 1

Reflect on Growth

Growth often becomes visible only when you pause long enough to notice it. Today invites you to reflect on how you have changed, learned, or adapted over time. Awareness deepens understanding.

Reflecting on growth does not require comparison or evaluation. It means noticing progress that may have occurred quietly. This recognition supports clarity.

As you move through the day, notice moments that reveal how far you have come. Allow yourself to acknowledge that growth. Reflection strengthens focus.

Growth becomes clearer through awareness. It builds confidence. Focus feels grounded.

SEPTEMBER 2

Reassess Priorities

Priorities can shift as circumstances and understanding change. Today invites you to gently reassess what currently deserves your attention and energy. Reflection supports alignment.

Reassessing priorities does not require immediate decisions or dramatic change. It means noticing where time and effort feel well spent. This awareness supports focus.

As you move through the day, notice which priorities feel most meaningful now. Allow yourself to adjust without pressure. Focus grows through honesty.

Clear priorities reduce distraction. They guide attention. Focus becomes intentional.

SEPTEMBER 3

Focus on Meaning

Meaning often provides deeper motivation than obligation alone. Today invites you to notice where meaning already exists in your daily life. Awareness restores purpose.

Focusing on meaning does not require grand answers or long-term plans. It means recognizing what feels worthwhile in this moment. This recognition supports clarity.

As you move through the day, notice activities or interactions that feel meaningful. Allow yourself to engage with them fully. Focus strengthens through purpose.

Meaning anchors attention. It sustains energy. Focus becomes fulfilling.

SEPTEMBER 4

Simplify Commitments

Commitments can accumulate until they diffuse attention and energy. Today invites you to notice which commitments truly require your focus. Simplification restores clarity.

Simplifying commitments does not mean neglecting responsibility. It means choosing where your energy has the greatest impact. This discernment supports focus.

As you move through the day, notice commitments that feel heavy or unnecessary. Allow yourself to adjust where possible. Focus responds to simplicity.

Simplified commitments reduce strain. They preserve attention. Focus becomes manageable.

SEPTEMBER 5

Recenter Attention

Attention naturally drifts when demands multiply. Today invites you to recenter your focus gently throughout the day. Awareness restores steadiness.

Recentering attention does not require constant correction. It means noticing when focus wanders and returning without judgment. This practice supports clarity.

As you move through the day, notice moments when you come back to what matters. Allow yourself to remain briefly. Focus deepens through repetition.

Recentered attention feels calm. It reduces overwhelm. Focus becomes stable.

SEPTEMBER 6

Learn From Experience

Experience often offers guidance that cannot be gained through planning alone. Today invites you to reflect on what recent experiences have taught you. Awareness transforms experience into insight.

Learning from experience does not require judgment or regret. It means noticing patterns, responses, and outcomes with curiosity. This reflection supports clarity.

As you move through the day, notice moments when past experience informs your choices. Allow yourself to trust that learning. Focus strengthens through understanding.

Experience becomes wisdom when acknowledged. It guides direction. Focus feels informed.

SEPTEMBER 7

Choose Intentional Focus

Focus becomes more effective when it is chosen rather than imposed. Today invites you to notice where your attention is most purposefully directed. Intention restores clarity.

Choosing intentional focus does not require rigid concentration. It means aligning attention with what matters most right now. This alignment supports steadiness.

As you move through the day, notice moments when you intentionally direct your focus. Allow yourself to remain with that choice. Focus deepens through intention.

Intentional focus reduces distraction. It clarifies effort. Focus becomes purposeful.

SEPTEMBER 8

Release Mental Clutter

Mental clutter can quietly drain attention and energy. Today invites you to notice thoughts that repeat without adding clarity. Awareness creates space.

Releasing mental clutter does not mean stopping thoughts entirely. It means allowing unnecessary mental noise to pass without engagement. This release supports focus.

As you move through the day, notice moments when your mind feels crowded. Allow yourself to let some thoughts go. Focus responds to openness.

Clear mental space supports attention. It reduces strain. Focus becomes lighter.

SEPTEMBER 9

Reconnect With Purpose

Purpose often becomes clearer when you pause long enough to notice it. Today invites you to reconnect with what motivates and guides you beneath routine. Reflection restores direction.

Reconnecting with purpose does not require redefining your life or goals. It means noticing what continues to feel meaningful. This awareness supports focus.

As you move through the day, notice moments when purpose feels present. Allow yourself to align with it gently. Focus strengthens through meaning.

Purpose anchors effort. It sustains attention. Focus becomes fulfilling.

SEPTEMBER 10

Strengthen Concentration

Concentration develops through practice rather than force. Today invites you to notice how sustained attention feels when it is supported rather than strained. Awareness builds steadiness.

Strengthening concentration does not require long periods of intense focus. It means choosing to stay with one task or thought for a little longer. This practice supports clarity.

As you move through the day, notice moments when concentration feels natural. Allow yourself to continue without interruption. Focus grows through presence.

Concentration supports effectiveness. It reduces fragmentation. Focus becomes steady.

SEPTEMBER 11

Align With Values

Values quietly guide decisions even when they are not named. Today invites you to notice where your actions align with what matters most to you. Awareness restores clarity.

Aligning with values does not require perfection or constant self-monitoring. It means recognizing moments when choices reflect your principles. This recognition supports focus.

As you move through the day, notice when your actions feel congruent and grounded. Allow yourself to acknowledge that alignment. Focus strengthens through integrity.

Values provide direction. They reduce confusion. Focus becomes anchored.

SEPTEMBER 12

Reflect Kindly

Reflection is most useful when it is gentle rather than critical. Today invites you to look back with kindness instead of judgment. Compassion supports insight.

Reflecting kindly does not mean ignoring mistakes or challenges. It means allowing understanding to replace harsh evaluation. This approach preserves clarity.

As you move through the day, notice moments when self-judgment arises during reflection. Allow yourself to soften your perspective. Focus grows through kindness.

Kind reflection supports learning. It protects motivation. Focus remains steady.

SEPTEMBER 13

Renew Direction

Direction can evolve as understanding deepens. Today invites you to notice where subtle shifts are guiding you forward. Awareness supports adjustment.

Renewing direction does not require abandoning past efforts. It means allowing insight to refine your path. This refinement strengthens focus.

As you move through the day, notice moments when clarity about next steps appears. Allow yourself to follow that guidance gently. Focus responds to alignment.

Renewed direction feels purposeful. It reduces hesitation. Focus becomes confident.

SEPTEMBER 14

Stay Focused Today

Focus often feels most manageable when approached one day at a time. Today invites you to bring attention back to what matters now. Presence restores steadiness.

Staying focused today does not require rigid discipline. It means choosing to return attention when it wanders. This practice supports clarity.

As you move through the day, notice moments when you refocus successfully. Allow yourself to recognize that effort. Focus strengthens through repetition.

Daily focus builds momentum. It reduces overwhelm. Focus becomes reliable.

SEPTEMBER 15

Reduce Distractions

Distractions can quietly dilute attention and energy. Today invites you to notice what pulls your focus away unnecessarily. Awareness restores clarity.

Reducing distractions does not require eliminating stimulation entirely. It means choosing what deserves your attention. This choice supports focus.

As you move through the day, notice moments when distractions arise. Allow yourself to disengage gently. Focus responds to intention.

Fewer distractions preserve energy. They support depth. Focus becomes sustained.

SEPTEMBER 16

Practice Mental Clarity

Mental clarity allows thoughts to settle into order without force. Today invites you to notice how clarity feels when the mind is given space. Awareness restores focus.

Practicing mental clarity does not require eliminating thoughts. It means allowing attention to rest on what is most relevant. This approach supports steadiness.

As you move through the day, notice moments when your thinking feels clear and unburdened. Allow yourself to remain there briefly. Focus grows through simplicity.

Mental clarity reduces strain. It supports decision-making. Focus becomes calm.

SEPTEMBER 17

Choose Depth Over Speed

Speed can scatter attention and dilute meaning. Today invites you to choose depth by slowing enough to engage fully. Depth strengthens focus.

Choosing depth over speed does not mean resisting efficiency. It means allowing quality to guide pace. This choice supports clarity.

As you move through the day, notice moments when slowing down improves understanding. Allow yourself to continue at that pace. Focus deepens through presence.

Depth enriches experience. It reduces error. Focus becomes intentional.

SEPTEMBER 18

Honor Focused Energy

Focused energy is a valuable resource that deserves protection. Today invites you to notice where your energy is being used most effectively. Awareness restores balance.

Honoring focused energy does not require constant productivity. It means respecting periods of concentration and rest. This respect supports focus.

As you move through the day, notice moments when your energy feels aligned with your attention. Allow yourself to protect that alignment. Focus grows through care.

Focused energy supports clarity. It sustains effort. Focus becomes sustainable.

SEPTEMBER 19

Clarify What's Next

Clarity about next steps often emerges through reflection rather than pressure. Today invites you to notice where understanding is already forming. Awareness guides direction.

Clarifying what is next does not require complete plans. It means recognizing the next reasonable step. This recognition supports focus.

As you move through the day, notice moments when direction feels clearer. Allow yourself to trust that guidance. Focus strengthens through trust.

Clear direction reduces hesitation. It supports movement. Focus becomes confident.

SEPTEMBER 20

End the Month Clear

As the month nears its close, today invites you to notice how reflection and focus have shaped your attention. Awareness allows clarity to integrate. Ending gently supports continuity.

Ending the month clear does not require summary or evaluation. It means acknowledging moments of insight and alignment. Recognition strengthens clarity.

As you move through the day, notice what feels clearer than before. Allow yourself to honor that shift. Focus carries forward naturally.

Clear endings feel grounded. They prepare what comes next. Focus remains steady.

SEPTEMBER 21

Carry Insight Forward

Insight becomes most valuable when it continues to inform daily choices. Today invites you to notice which realizations from recent reflection feel worth carrying forward. Continuity supports clarity.

Carrying insight forward does not require constant analysis. It means allowing understanding to quietly influence how you respond and decide. This integration supports focus.

As you move through the day, notice moments when insight guides your actions naturally. Allow yourself to trust that influence. Focus grows through integration.

Insight carried forward feels steady. It reduces confusion. Focus becomes grounded.

SEPTEMBER 22

Stay Mindfully Focused

Mindful focus allows attention to remain present without strain. Today invites you to notice how awareness supports steadiness when distractions arise. Mindfulness restores clarity.

Staying mindfully focused does not mean rigid concentration. It means gently returning attention when it drifts. This practice supports sustainable focus.

As you move through the day, notice moments when mindfulness anchors your attention. Allow yourself to remain there briefly. Focus deepens through awareness.

Mindful focus reduces fatigue. It supports balance. Focus becomes calm.

SEPTEMBER 23

Review Without Pressure

Reviewing past choices can offer clarity when done without judgment. Today invites you to look back with curiosity rather than urgency. Ease supports insight.

Reviewing without pressure does not require fixing or correcting everything. It means noticing patterns and learning gently. This approach preserves focus.

As you move through the day, notice moments when reflection feels neutral rather than heavy. Allow yourself to remain there. Focus responds to kindness.

Gentle review supports learning. It protects motivation. Focus stays steady.

SEPTEMBER 24

Trust Thoughtful Progress

Progress often unfolds through steady, thoughtful steps rather than rapid change. Today invites you to trust the pace of your development. Patience supports focus.

Trusting thoughtful progress does not mean resisting growth. It means allowing understanding to guide movement. This trust reduces pressure.

As you move through the day, notice moments when progress feels subtle yet real. Allow yourself to acknowledge that movement. Focus strengthens through patience.

Thoughtful progress builds confidence. It reduces strain. Focus remains consistent.

SEPTEMBER 25

Focus on Essentials

Essentials provide clarity when attention feels scattered. Today invites you to notice what truly requires your focus right now. Simplicity restores direction.

Focusing on essentials does not require minimizing complexity. It means prioritizing what matters most in this moment. This discernment supports focus.

As you move through the day, notice where attention feels best placed. Allow yourself to let go of what is nonessential. Focus grows through simplicity.

Essentials anchor attention. They reduce overwhelm. Focus becomes clear.

SEPTEMBER 26

Refine Your Focus

Focus becomes clearer when it is refined rather than expanded. Today invites you to notice where narrowing attention improves clarity and effectiveness. Refinement supports steadiness.

Refining your focus does not require eliminating interests or possibilities. It means choosing what deserves your attention right now. This choice supports direction.

As you move through the day, notice moments when simplifying focus feels supportive. Allow yourself to commit to fewer priorities. Focus grows through precision.

Refined focus reduces noise. It preserves energy. Attention becomes intentional.

SEPTEMBER 27

Trust Quiet Insight

Insight often arrives quietly rather than dramatically. Today invites you to notice subtle understanding that emerges without force. Listening supports clarity.

Trusting quiet insight does not require immediate action. It means allowing understanding to settle before responding. This patience supports focus.

As you move through the day, notice moments when insight feels subtle but steady. Allow yourself to trust that awareness. Focus strengthens through listening.

Quiet insight guides gently. It reduces confusion. Focus becomes assured.

SEPTEMBER 28

Let Clarity Settle

Clarity deepens when it is given time to settle rather than rushed into action. Today invites you to allow understanding to rest within you. Settling supports focus.

Letting clarity settle does not mean delaying progress. It means allowing certainty to form naturally. This approach reduces pressure.

As you move through the day, notice moments when clarity feels calm rather than urgent. Allow yourself to remain there briefly. Focus grows through patience.

Settled clarity feels grounded. It supports confidence. Focus becomes stable.

SEPTEMBER 29

Prepare for What's Ahead

Preparation becomes meaningful when guided by reflection rather than anxiety. Today invites you to consider what lies ahead with calm attention. Awareness supports readiness.

Preparing for what is ahead does not require detailed plans. It means noticing what feels relevant to consider next. This awareness supports focus.

As you move through the day, notice moments when preparation feels supportive rather than stressful. Allow yourself to respond thoughtfully. Focus strengthens through foresight.

Thoughtful preparation reduces uncertainty. It supports direction. Focus remains clear.

SEPTEMBER 30

Close the Month Focused

As September comes to a close, today invites you to notice how reflection and focus have shaped your attention and priorities. Integration allows clarity to remain. Ending gently supports continuity.

Closing the month focused does not require evaluation or summary. It means acknowledging moments of insight, steadiness, and alignment. Recognition strengthens focus.

As you move through the day, notice what feels clearer or more intentional than before. Allow yourself to honor that awareness. Focus carries forward naturally.

Focused endings feel grounded. They prepare the next phase. Attention remains aligned.

OCTOBER

Acceptance & Ease

October invites a gentler way of moving through life, one that emphasizes acceptance rather than effort and ease rather than struggle. This month centers on allowing experience to unfold without constant resistance or control. Acceptance becomes a source of relief.

Ease is not something that must be earned or justified. It emerges when you stop fighting what is already present and allow yourself to soften. Acceptance creates space for calm.

As you move through October, let acceptance guide your responses and ease shape your pace. Allow softness to replace urgency. Relief grows through allowing.

OCTOBER 1

Accept Yourself Fully

Acceptance begins with how you relate to yourself in this moment. Today invites you to notice parts of yourself that seek permission to exist as they are. Acceptance restores ease.

Accepting yourself fully does not require approval of everything you feel or do. It means allowing your humanity without constant correction. This allowance softens inner tension.

As you move through the day, notice moments when self-judgment appears. Allow yourself to replace it with understanding. Ease grows through self-acceptance.

Self-acceptance creates inner safety. It reduces resistance. Ease becomes accessible.

OCTOBER 2

Release Resistance

Resistance often appears as tension, frustration, or mental struggle. Today invites you to notice where you are pushing against what already exists. Awareness restores ease.

Releasing resistance does not mean giving up or disengaging. It means allowing reality to be acknowledged before responding. This acknowledgment softens effort.

As you move through the day, notice moments when resistance tightens your body or thoughts. Allow yourself to relax that grip gently. Ease responds to release.

Reduced resistance conserves energy. It restores clarity. Ease feels natural.

OCTOBER 3

Allow Natural Flow

Life often moves more smoothly when you stop interrupting its rhythm. Today invites you to notice where things are unfolding without effort. Flow supports ease.

Allowing natural flow does not mean avoiding responsibility. It means trusting timing and movement rather than forcing outcomes. This trust restores calm.

As you move through the day, notice moments when you let things progress naturally. Allow yourself to stay with that flow. Ease grows through trust.

Natural flow reduces strain. It aligns effort. Ease becomes steady.

OCTOBER 4

Practice Emotional Acceptance

Emotions come and go whether they are welcomed or resisted. Today invites you to allow feelings to exist without trying to change them. Acceptance supports ease.

Practicing emotional acceptance does not require liking or approving of emotions. It means letting them be present without adding struggle. This allowance softens experience.

As you move through the day, notice emotions as they arise. Allow yourself to acknowledge them without reaction. Ease grows through acceptance.

Accepted emotions settle naturally. They lose intensity. Ease follows honesty.

OCTOBER 5

Ease Into Moments

Moments feel lighter when you enter them without tension. Today invites you to slow your approach and allow ease to guide your transitions. Gentleness supports calm.

Easing into moments does not require extra time or preparation. It means softening your pace mentally and physically. This softness restores balance.

As you move through the day, notice how you enter tasks or conversations. Allow yourself to arrive with ease. Calm responds to gentleness.

Gentle entry reduces strain. It supports presence. Ease becomes habitual.

OCTOBER 6

Welcome Imperfection

Imperfection is a natural part of living and learning. Today invites you to notice where striving for flawlessness creates unnecessary tension. Acceptance restores ease.

Welcoming imperfection does not mean lowering standards or avoiding growth. It means allowing room for error without self-criticism. This permission softens effort.

As you move through the day, notice moments when imperfection appears. Allow yourself to meet it with understanding. Ease grows through compassion.

Imperfection humanizes experience. It reduces pressure. Ease becomes more accessible.

OCTOBER 7

Choose Softness

Softness allows you to meet life without armor. Today invites you to notice where gentleness could replace rigidity. Softness supports ease.

Choosing softness does not mean avoiding strength or clarity. It means allowing your responses to be flexible rather than forceful. This choice reduces strain.

As you move through the day, notice moments when you can soften your tone or pace. Allow yourself to do so intentionally. Ease responds to gentleness.

Softness calms the body. It relaxes the mind. Ease feels supportive.

OCTOBER 8

Let Go Gently

Letting go often happens gradually rather than all at once. Today invites you to release what feels heavy with patience and care. Gentleness preserves ease.

Letting go gently does not require resolution or closure. It means loosening your grip on what no longer serves you. This release creates space.

As you move through the day, notice moments when holding on feels unnecessary. Allow yourself to soften your attachment. Ease grows through release.

Gentle letting go restores balance. It reduces tension. Ease follows lightness.

OCTOBER 9

Practice Letting Be

Some experiences require acceptance rather than action. Today invites you to practice letting things be as they are. Allowing supports ease.

Practicing letting be does not mean passivity or avoidance. It means recognizing when intervention is unnecessary. This recognition reduces effort.

As you move through the day, notice situations that can remain unchanged. Allow yourself to stop trying to fix them. Ease grows through allowance.

Letting be calms inner resistance. It restores peace. Ease becomes steady.

OCTOBER 10

Accept Change Calmly

Change can feel unsettling when it is resisted. Today invites you to meet change with calm awareness. Acceptance supports ease.

Accepting change calmly does not require liking uncertainty. It means acknowledging shifts without panic or control. This acceptance steadies response.

As you move through the day, notice changes as they occur. Allow yourself to respond with openness rather than tension. Ease grows through trust.

Calm acceptance stabilizes emotion. It reduces fear. Ease accompanies adaptation.

OCTOBER 11

Trust Life's Rhythm

Life often unfolds according to rhythms that cannot be rushed or controlled. Today invites you to notice where timing is already supporting you. Trust restores ease.

Trusting life's rhythm does not mean waiting passively or giving up effort. It means recognizing when pushing creates resistance rather than progress. This awareness softens strain.

As you move through the day, notice moments when things unfold naturally. Allow yourself to trust that timing. Ease grows through alignment.

Natural rhythm steadies movement. It reduces urgency. Ease becomes reassuring.

OCTOBER 12

Stop Forcing Outcomes

Forcing outcomes can create exhaustion and frustration. Today invites you to notice where effort has turned into strain. Awareness restores ease.

Stopping the need to force outcomes does not mean abandoning goals. It means allowing processes to unfold without constant pressure. This shift supports calm.

As you move through the day, notice moments when you tighten around results. Allow yourself to loosen that grip. Ease responds to release.

Reduced force conserves energy. It restores clarity. Ease feels natural.

OCTOBER 13

Allow Space for Ease

Ease requires space to emerge and be felt. Today invites you to notice where space can soften your experience. Openness supports relief.

Allowing space for ease does not require removing all responsibility. It means creating small pauses or gentler transitions. This openness restores balance.

As you move through the day, notice moments when space feels supportive. Allow yourself to stay there briefly. Ease grows through permission.

Space reduces tension. It restores calm. Ease becomes available.

OCTOBER 14

Choose Grace Over Struggle

Grace allows movement without constant resistance. Today invites you to notice where struggle has become habitual. Choice restores ease.

Choosing grace over struggle does not mean avoiding effort. It means responding with acceptance rather than resistance. This approach supports calm.

As you move through the day, notice moments when grace feels possible. Allow yourself to respond with softness. Ease grows through grace.

Grace simplifies experience. It reduces effort. Ease becomes sustainable.

OCTOBER 15

Relax Expectations

Expectations can quietly create pressure and disappointment. Today invites you to notice where expectations could be softened. Relaxation restores ease.

Relaxing expectations does not mean lowering standards or disengaging. It means allowing flexibility in how outcomes unfold. This flexibility supports calm.

As you move through the day, notice moments when expectations tighten your experience. Allow yourself to loosen them gently. Ease responds to openness.

Relaxed expectations reduce strain. They restore presence. Ease feels natural.

OCTOBER 16

Let Things Unfold

Life often resolves itself when given enough time and space. Today invites you to notice where patience allows clarity to emerge naturally. Allowing supports ease.

Letting things unfold does not mean disengaging or ignoring responsibility. It means trusting that not everything requires immediate intervention. This trust softens effort.

As you move through the day, notice moments when waiting feels supportive. Allow yourself to remain present without rushing. Ease grows through patience.

Unfolding restores balance. It reduces urgency. Ease becomes reassuring.

OCTOBER 17

Trust the Process

Processes develop through stages that cannot be skipped. Today invites you to notice where progress is happening even if outcomes are not visible yet. Trust restores calm.

Trusting the process does not require certainty or optimism. It means staying engaged without demanding immediate results. This steadiness supports ease.

As you move through the day, notice moments when progress feels gradual. Allow yourself to trust that movement is occurring. Ease grows through confidence.

Process trust reduces frustration. It sustains effort. Ease remains steady.

OCTOBER 18

Accept What's Present

Acceptance begins with acknowledging what is happening right now. Today invites you to notice where resisting the present moment creates tension. Acceptance restores ease.

Accepting what is present does not mean approval or resignation. It means allowing reality to be seen clearly before responding. This honesty softens strain.

As you move through the day, notice moments when acceptance feels possible. Allow yourself to relax into that awareness. Ease grows through truth.

Present acceptance stabilizes emotion. It reduces conflict. Ease feels grounded.

OCTOBER 19

Move With Ease

Movement feels lighter when it is guided by awareness rather than pressure. Today invites you to notice how ease can shape both action and rest. Gentleness supports flow.

Moving with ease does not mean slowing everything down. It means adjusting effort so that movement feels sustainable. This adjustment preserves energy.

As you move through the day, notice when ease influences your pace. Allow yourself to follow that guidance. Ease grows through alignment.

Easeful movement reduces strain. It supports balance. Flow becomes natural.

OCTOBER 20

Stay Open and Soft

Openness allows experience to be met without armor or resistance. Today invites you to notice where softness can replace defensiveness. Softness supports ease.

Staying open and soft does not mean losing boundaries or clarity. It means remaining receptive while grounded. This balance preserves calm.

As you move through the day, notice moments when openness feels safe. Allow yourself to remain there. Ease grows through receptivity.

Soft openness calms the nervous system. It reduces tension. Ease feels supportive.

OCTOBER 21

End the Month At Ease

As the month begins to settle toward its close, today invites you to notice where ease has quietly entered your experience. Reflection allows that ease to be recognized rather than overlooked. Awareness replaces effort.

Ending the month at ease does not require everything to feel resolved or perfect. It means acknowledging moments when softness replaced struggle. This recognition deepens calm.

As you move through the day, notice where your body or mind feels more relaxed than before. Allow yourself to honor that shift. Ease grows through acknowledgment.

Easeful endings integrate experience. They reduce tension. Calm feels embodied.

OCTOBER 22

Carry Acceptance Forward

Acceptance becomes most supportive when it continues beyond a single moment. Today invites you to notice which forms of acceptance you want to carry forward into daily life. Continuity supports ease.

Carrying acceptance forward does not mean tolerating what causes harm. It means allowing reality to be met honestly before choosing how to respond. This honesty preserves calm.

As you move through the day, notice moments when acceptance softens your reaction. Allow yourself to continue that approach. Ease grows through consistency.

Sustained acceptance reduces resistance. It conserves energy. Ease becomes natural.

OCTOBER 23

Ease Is Allowed

Ease often feels restricted by habit or belief. Today invites you to recognize that ease is permitted without justification. Permission restores relief.

Allowing ease does not mean neglecting responsibility or purpose. It means releasing the idea that difficulty is required. This release supports calm.

As you move through the day, notice moments when ease feels possible. Allow yourself to accept it without explanation. Ease grows through permission.

Allowed ease settles deeply. It reduces strain. Calm becomes accessible.

OCTOBER 24

Breathe Into Allowing

Breath can guide you into acceptance without effort. Today invites you to use breathing as a way to soften resistance and invite allowing. Awareness restores ease.

Breathing into allowing does not require technique or control. It means letting breath move naturally while attention softens. This approach supports calm.

As you move through the day, notice moments when tension arises. Allow your breath to invite release. Ease grows through presence.

Breath anchors acceptance. It calms the body. Ease becomes embodied.

OCTOBER 25

Choose Peace Today

Peace often emerges from choices made moment by moment. Today invites you to notice where peace is available through acceptance and ease. Awareness restores calm.

Choosing peace today does not mean avoiding difficulty. It means responding without adding unnecessary struggle. This choice supports steadiness.

As you move through the day, notice moments when peace feels accessible. Allow yourself to choose it gently. Ease grows through intention.

Peaceful choices reduce tension. They support clarity. Calm becomes sustainable.

OCTOBER 26

Let Go Again

Letting go often needs to happen more than once. Today invites you to notice where something you released earlier has quietly returned. Awareness restores ease.

Letting go again does not mean failure or regression. It means honoring the ongoing nature of release. This understanding softens frustration.

As you move through the day, notice what feels ready to be released once more. Allow yourself to loosen your grip gently. Ease grows through repetition.

Repeated release lightens experience. It reduces attachment. Ease feels renewed.

OCTOBER 27

Rest in Acceptance

Acceptance can become a place of rest rather than effort. Today invites you to notice how allowing things to be creates calm. Rest supports ease.

Resting in acceptance does not require disengagement or passivity. It means stopping the internal struggle against what exists. This rest restores balance.

As you move through the day, notice moments when acceptance feels settling. Allow yourself to remain there. Ease grows through stillness.

Acceptance offers relief. It calms the nervous system. Ease feels supportive.

OCTOBER 28

Soften Your Pace

Pace influences how experience is felt in the body and mind. Today invites you to notice where slowing slightly could bring relief. Softness restores ease.

Softening your pace does not mean delaying progress. It means adjusting speed to match capacity. This adjustment supports balance.

As you move through the day, notice moments when rushing creates tension. Allow yourself to ease your pace gently. Ease grows through alignment.

A softer pace reduces strain. It preserves energy. Ease becomes sustainable.

OCTOBER 29

Trust Ease to Guide You

Ease can act as a guide when decisions feel unclear. Today invites you to notice which choices feel lighter and more natural. Trust restores calm.

Trusting ease to guide you does not mean avoiding responsibility. It means allowing comfort and alignment to inform direction. This guidance supports clarity.

As you move through the day, notice moments when ease influences your choices. Allow yourself to follow that signal. Ease grows through trust.

Ease guides gently. It reduces resistance. Calm becomes intuitive.

OCTOBER 30

Allow Gentle Endings

Endings can feel softer when approached with acceptance. Today invites you to notice how allowing closure gently supports peace. Gentleness restores ease.

Allowing gentle endings does not require resolution of every detail. It means honoring completion without urgency. This approach preserves calm.

As you move through the day, notice moments that feel ready to conclude. Allow yourself to let them end naturally. Ease grows through closure.

Gentle endings bring relief. They reduce tension. Ease settles naturally.

OCTOBER 31

Close the Month With Ease

As October comes to a close, today invites you to reflect on how acceptance and ease have shaped your experience. Integration allows calm to remain. Ending softly supports continuity.

Closing the month with ease does not require summary or evaluation. It means acknowledging moments when allowing replaced struggle. Recognition deepens peace.

As you move through the day, notice what feels softer or lighter than before. Allow yourself to honor that shift. Ease carries forward naturally.

Easeful closures feel grounded. They prepare the next phase. Calm remains accessible.

NOVEMBER

Gratitude & Connection

November invites attention toward what supports you and the relationships that quietly shape your life. This month focuses on gratitude that feels grounded and connection that grows through presence rather than obligation. Appreciation becomes relational.

Gratitude here is not forced or performative. It is noticed slowly through lived experience and shared moments. Connection deepens when it is allowed to be sincere.

As you move through November, let gratitude soften your perspective and connection steady your sense of belonging. Allow appreciation to feel mutual. Meaning grows through relationship.

NOVEMBER 1

Notice Support Around You

Support often exists in ways that are easy to overlook when attention is focused inward or ahead. Today invites you to notice where support already surrounds you. Awareness restores connection.

Noticing support does not require comparing or evaluating relationships. It means acknowledging presence, reliability, or care where it exists. This recognition deepens gratitude.

As you move through the day, notice gestures or systems that support you quietly. Allow yourself to acknowledge them internally. Gratitude grows through awareness.

Support creates stability. It reduces isolation. Connection feels reinforced.

NOVEMBER 2

Appreciate Simple Comforts

Simple comforts can ground you during ordinary moments. Today invites you to notice small sources of ease or warmth in your day. Attention restores appreciation.

Appreciating simple comforts does not require creating special circumstances. It means recognizing what already provides reassurance or calm. This noticing supports gratitude.

As you move through the day, notice physical or emotional comforts that feel supportive. Allow yourself to linger briefly. Gratitude grows through presence.

Simple comforts soften experience. They provide steadiness. Connection to the moment deepens.

NOVEMBER 3

Express Quiet Gratitude

Gratitude does not always need to be spoken aloud. Today invites you to express appreciation internally and sincerely. Quiet acknowledgment supports connection.

Expressing quiet gratitude does not mean withholding appreciation from others. It means allowing gratitude to exist even when unspoken. This presence deepens awareness.

As you move through the day, notice moments when appreciation arises naturally. Allow yourself to hold that feeling gently. Gratitude strengthens through sincerity.

Quiet gratitude feels grounding. It stabilizes emotion. Connection grows inwardly.

NOVEMBER 4

Acknowledge Small Blessings

Small blessings often pass unnoticed when attention is elsewhere. Today invites you to acknowledge modest positives without minimizing them. Recognition supports gratitude.

Acknowledging small blessings does not require constant scanning for positivity. It means allowing appreciation to arise naturally. This allowance sustains balance.

As you move through the day, notice moments that feel helpful or kind. Allow yourself to recognize them. Gratitude grows through acknowledgment.

Small blessings accumulate quietly. They support resilience. Connection to life deepens.

NOVEMBER 5

Strengthen Meaningful Connections

Meaningful connections grow through consistent presence rather than intensity. Today invites you to notice which relationships feel supportive and genuine. Awareness strengthens bonds.

Strengthening connections does not require constant interaction. It means valuing trust, care, and understanding where they exist. This valuing supports gratitude.

As you move through the day, notice moments of connection that feel sincere. Allow yourself to engage with care. Gratitude deepens through relationship.

Meaningful connections offer grounding. They support belonging. Appreciation becomes shared.

NOVEMBER 6

Appreciate Shared Moments

Shared moments often hold meaning long after they pass. Today invites you to notice interactions or experiences that feel quietly significant. Awareness deepens gratitude.

Appreciating shared moments does not require them to be dramatic or rare. It means recognizing presence, exchange, and mutual attention. This recognition strengthens connection.

As you move through the day, notice moments when time is shared comfortably. Allow yourself to value those moments. Gratitude grows through shared experience.

Shared moments create memory. They reinforce belonging. Connection feels affirmed.

NOVEMBER 7

Offer Kind Presence

Presence can be one of the most meaningful gifts you offer another person. Today invites you to show up with attentiveness and care. Kindness supports connection.

Offering kind presence does not require advice or solutions. It means being available, listening, and allowing space. This availability fosters trust.

As you move through the day, notice opportunities to be present without distraction. Allow yourself to offer that presence fully. Gratitude grows through sincerity.

Kind presence builds safety. It strengthens relationships. Connection deepens naturally.

NOVEMBER 8

Receive Appreciation

Receiving appreciation can feel uncomfortable when humility or habit encourages deflection. Today invites you to accept appreciation without minimizing it. Acceptance supports gratitude.

Receiving appreciation does not mean seeking validation. It means allowing acknowledgment to be received fully. This openness strengthens connection.

As you move through the day, notice moments when appreciation is offered. Allow yourself to accept it without explanation. Gratitude grows through reception.

Accepted appreciation reinforces worth. It deepens connection. Balance is restored.

NOVEMBER 9

Practice Thankful Awareness

Thankful awareness involves noticing gratitude as it naturally arises. Today invites you to stay attentive to moments that evoke appreciation. Awareness supports connection.

Practicing thankful awareness does not require constant positivity. It means allowing gratitude to coexist with complexity. This balance sustains sincerity.

As you move through the day, notice feelings of thankfulness as they appear. Allow yourself to acknowledge them gently. Gratitude grows through attention.

Thankful awareness stabilizes perspective. It grounds emotion. Connection feels supported.

NOVEMBER 10

Honor Support Systems

Support systems often function quietly in the background of daily life. Today invites you to recognize structures and people that provide stability. Recognition deepens gratitude.

Honoring support systems does not require formal acknowledgment. It means appreciating reliability and presence. This appreciation strengthens connection.

As you move through the day, notice systems or individuals that make life easier. Allow yourself to recognize their value. Gratitude grows through awareness.

Support systems create security. They reduce burden. Connection feels reliable.

NOVEMBER 11

Reach Out Gently

Reaching out can strengthen connection when it is done with care and sincerity. Today invites you to notice where gentle contact could support understanding or closeness. Awareness restores warmth.

Reaching out gently does not require long conversations or explanations. It means offering presence, a message, or a moment of attention. This gesture supports connection.

As you move through the day, notice moments when reaching out feels natural. Allow yourself to act without pressure. Gratitude grows through openness.

Gentle outreach reduces distance. It fosters trust. Connection becomes more accessible.

NOVEMBER 12

Connect Without Expectations

Expectations can quietly shape how connection feels. Today invites you to engage with others without anticipating specific outcomes. Ease supports authenticity.

Connecting without expectations does not mean disengagement or indifference. It means allowing interactions to unfold naturally. This openness deepens gratitude.

As you move through the day, notice moments when you release expectations. Allow yourself to stay present. Connection grows through freedom.

Expectation-free connection feels lighter. It reduces strain. Gratitude becomes sincere.

NOVEMBER 13

Appreciate Emotional Safety

Emotional safety allows honesty, ease, and trust to develop. Today invites you to notice where you feel understood or accepted. Awareness deepens gratitude.

Appreciating emotional safety does not require constant reassurance. It means recognizing environments or relationships where you can be yourself. This recognition supports connection.

As you move through the day, notice moments when emotional safety is present. Allow yourself to value those spaces. Gratitude grows through acknowledgment.

Emotional safety fosters belonging. It supports well-being. Connection feels secure.

NOVEMBER 14

Value Shared Humanity

Shared humanity connects people through common experience. Today invites you to notice similarities rather than differences. Awareness softens perspective.

Valuing shared humanity does not mean minimizing individuality. It means recognizing common emotions, needs, and challenges. This recognition supports compassion.

As you move through the day, notice moments when shared experience becomes visible. Allow yourself to respond with understanding. Gratitude grows through empathy.

Shared humanity builds compassion. It reduces isolation. Connection feels inclusive.

NOVEMBER 15

Practice Listening Fully

Listening creates space for understanding and respect. Today invites you to listen without planning a response or solution. Attention strengthens connection.

Practicing full listening does not require silence or agreement. It means offering your full presence. This presence deepens gratitude.

As you move through the day, notice moments when you listen attentively. Allow yourself to remain engaged. Connection grows through attention.

Full listening fosters trust. It deepens relationships. Gratitude becomes relational.

NOVEMBER 16

Express Appreciation Clearly

Clear appreciation helps others feel seen and valued. Today invites you to express gratitude in ways that feel sincere and grounded. Clarity strengthens connection.

Expressing appreciation clearly does not require elaborate language or grand gestures. It means communicating thanks in a way that reflects genuine feeling. This honesty supports gratitude.

As you move through the day, notice moments when appreciation feels appropriate to express. Allow yourself to share it without hesitation. Gratitude grows through expression.

Clear appreciation builds trust. It affirms connection. Gratitude becomes shared.

NOVEMBER 17

Nurture Trust

Trust develops through consistency, honesty, and presence over time. Today invites you to notice where trust already exists in your relationships. Awareness strengthens bonds.

Nurturing trust does not require immediate vulnerability or disclosure. It means continuing to show up in ways that feel reliable and respectful. This steadiness supports connection.

As you move through the day, notice moments when trust is reinforced through small actions. Allow yourself to value those moments. Gratitude grows through reliability.

Trust provides emotional safety. It deepens connection. Gratitude feels secure.

NOVEMBER 18

Stay Connected Kindly

Connection thrives when it is approached with kindness rather than obligation. Today invites you to engage with others in ways that feel warm and respectful. Kindness sustains relationships.

Staying connected kindly does not require constant communication or availability. It means offering care without pressure. This approach supports gratitude.

As you move through the day, notice moments when kindness shapes your interactions. Allow yourself to remain gentle. Connection grows through compassion.

Kind connection reduces strain. It fosters ease. Gratitude becomes natural.

NOVEMBER 19

End the Month Grateful

As the month begins to draw toward its close, today invites you to reflect on gratitude that has been present throughout November. Reflection allows appreciation to settle. Awareness replaces urgency.

Ending the month grateful does not require listing or summarizing everything you appreciate. It means acknowledging the presence of gratitude itself. This acknowledgment deepens connection.

As you move through the day, notice feelings of appreciation as they arise. Allow yourself to rest in them. Gratitude carries forward through awareness.

Grateful endings feel grounding. They support continuity. Connection remains strong.

NOVEMBER 20

Carry Gratitude Forward

Gratitude becomes more meaningful when it continues beyond a single moment or month. Today invites you to notice which forms of appreciation you want to carry forward. Continuity supports connection.

Carrying gratitude forward does not require constant focus or effort. It means allowing appreciation to inform how you relate to others and yourself. This integration supports balance.

As you move through the day, notice moments when gratitude influences your perspective. Allow yourself to continue that orientation. Gratitude grows through consistency.

Sustained gratitude stabilizes emotion. It deepens relationships. Connection feels enduring.

NOVEMBER 21

Notice Everyday Gifts

Everyday gifts often appear quietly within routine moments. Today invites you to notice small, ordinary experiences that offer support or comfort. Awareness deepens gratitude.

Noticing everyday gifts does not require searching for positivity. It means allowing appreciation to arise naturally within what is already present. This recognition supports connection.

As you move through the day, notice moments that feel helpful, steady, or kind. Allow yourself to acknowledge them gently. Gratitude grows through attention.

Everyday gifts ground experience. They reduce striving. Connection to life deepens.

NOVEMBER 22

Choose Appreciation Daily

Appreciation becomes more meaningful when it is practiced consistently. Today invites you to choose appreciation as a daily orientation rather than an occasional response. Intention strengthens gratitude.

Choosing appreciation daily does not mean ignoring difficulty. It means allowing appreciation to coexist with complexity. This balance supports connection.

As you move through the day, notice moments when appreciation feels available. Allow yourself to choose it deliberately. Gratitude grows through practice.

Daily appreciation steadies perspective. It supports resilience. Connection feels sustained.

NOVEMBER 23

Strengthen Bonds Slowly

Strong bonds develop through time, patience, and presence. Today invites you to notice how gradual connection creates trust. Awareness restores appreciation.

Strengthening bonds slowly does not require constant interaction. It means valuing consistency and reliability. This approach supports gratitude.

As you move through the day, notice moments when connection deepens quietly. Allow yourself to appreciate that growth. Gratitude grows through patience.

Slow bonds feel secure. They reduce pressure. Connection becomes lasting.

NOVEMBER 24

Let Gratitude Ground You

Gratitude can anchor you during moments of uncertainty or transition. Today invites you to notice how appreciation brings steadiness. Awareness supports grounding.

Letting gratitude ground you does not require forcing positive thinking. It means allowing appreciation to stabilize your perspective. This grounding supports connection.

As you move through the day, notice moments when gratitude calms or centers you. Allow yourself to remain there briefly. Gratitude grows through grounding.

Grounded gratitude stabilizes emotion. It restores balance. Connection feels rooted.

NOVEMBER 25

Return to Appreciation

Appreciation can be returned to whenever attention drifts or becomes strained. Today invites you to notice how easily gratitude can be revisited. Awareness restores connection.

Returning to appreciation does not require changing circumstances. It means shifting attention gently toward what supports you. This shift sustains gratitude.

As you move through the day, notice moments when appreciation reappears naturally. Allow yourself to welcome it. Gratitude grows through return.

Appreciation remains accessible. It steadies perspective. Connection continues.

NOVEMBER 26

Deepen Appreciation

Appreciation can grow deeper when it is revisited with attention and care. Today invites you to notice how gratitude expands when you stay with it a little longer. Awareness enriches connection.

Deepening appreciation does not require intensity or emotional display. It means allowing gratitude to settle and become more felt. This presence strengthens meaning.

As you move through the day, notice moments when appreciation lingers. Allow yourself to remain with that feeling. Gratitude grows through depth.

Deep appreciation feels grounding. It stabilizes emotion. Connection becomes more meaningful.

NOVEMBER 27

Honor What Has Supported You

Support often becomes visible only in hindsight. Today invites you to honor what has carried you through recent days or seasons. Recognition strengthens gratitude.

Honoring support does not require perfection or constant reliance. It means acknowledging contributions, seen or unseen. This acknowledgment deepens connection.

As you move through the day, notice people, routines, or structures that have supported you. Allow yourself to honor their role. Gratitude grows through recognition.

Honored support reinforces trust. It builds appreciation. Connection feels affirmed.

NOVEMBER 28

Allow Gratitude to Soften You

Gratitude can soften emotional edges and reduce inner tension. Today invites you to notice how appreciation changes how you feel internally. Softness supports connection.

Allowing gratitude to soften you does not mean becoming passive or sentimental. It means letting appreciation relax your stance toward life. This relaxation restores balance.

As you move through the day, notice moments when gratitude eases emotional weight. Allow yourself to soften into that experience. Gratitude grows through ease.

Softened gratitude calms the nervous system. It restores openness. Connection feels gentler.

NOVEMBER 29

Prepare to Carry Connection Forward

Connection becomes sustainable when it is carried with intention. Today invites you to notice which forms of connection you want to preserve moving forward. Awareness supports continuity.

Preparing to carry connection forward does not require promises or obligation. It means valuing what feels meaningful enough to maintain. This valuing strengthens gratitude.

As you move through the day, notice relationships or practices you want to continue nurturing. Allow yourself to hold them with care. Gratitude grows through intention.

Sustained connection supports belonging. It stabilizes relationships. Appreciation remains active.

NOVEMBER 30

Close the Month Connected

As November comes to a close, today invites you to notice how gratitude and connection have shaped your experience. Integration allows appreciation to remain present. Ending gently supports continuity.

Closing the month connected does not require summary or evaluation. It means acknowledging moments of warmth, support, and shared presence. Recognition deepens meaning.

As you move through the day, notice what feels more connected than before. Allow yourself to honor that shift. Gratitude carries forward naturally.

Connected endings feel grounding. They reinforce belonging. Appreciation remains alive.

DECEMBER

Rest & Renewal

December invites a gradual slowing, offering space to rest, reflect, and release before something new begins. This period honors completion as much as beginning, allowing the year to settle fully before moving forward. Rest becomes purposeful rather than passive.

Renewal here is not rushed or forced. It unfolds through quiet reflection, intentional rest, and gentle closure. Wisdom accumulates when nothing is hurried.

As you move through December, allow yourself to rest deeply and reflect honestly. Let renewal emerge naturally. Completion and beginning coexist here.

DECEMBER 1

Slow the Pace

The end of the year often arrives with urgency and expectation. Today invites you to slow your pace deliberately, even when momentum pushes otherwise. Slowing restores balance.

Slowing the pace does not mean disengaging from life or responsibility. It means choosing a rhythm that supports steadiness rather than strain. This choice protects energy.

As you move through the day, notice moments when you rush unnecessarily. Allow yourself to soften your pace gently. Rest begins through intention.

A slower pace calms the body. It quiets the mind. Renewal feels possible.

DECEMBER 2

Create Space for Rest

Rest requires space in order to be felt and received. Today invites you to notice where small openings for rest already exist. Awareness restores permission.

Creating space for rest does not require long breaks or perfect conditions. It means allowing moments of pause within ordinary activity. This allowance supports renewal.

As you move through the day, notice opportunities to step back briefly. Allow yourself to take them without justification. Rest grows through permission.

Rested space restores clarity. It reduces fatigue. Renewal begins gently.

DECEMBER 3

Reflect on the Year

Reflection allows experience to be integrated rather than forgotten. Today invites you to look back on the year with openness rather than judgment. Awareness brings understanding.

Reflecting on the year does not require evaluating success or failure. It means noticing what shaped you, challenged you, and supported you. This reflection deepens wisdom.

As you move through the day, notice memories or themes that arise naturally. Allow yourself to acknowledge them gently. Insight grows through reflection.

Yearly reflection offers perspective. It clarifies meaning. Renewal becomes informed.

DECEMBER 4

Release What's Outgrown

Some patterns, beliefs, or expectations no longer serve who you are becoming. Today invites you to notice what feels ready to be released. Awareness restores lightness.

Releasing what is outgrown does not require dramatic action or resolution. It means loosening attachment to what no longer fits. This release supports rest.

As you move through the day, notice thoughts or habits that feel outdated. Allow yourself to let them go gently. Renewal grows through release.

Letting go creates space. It reduces inner weight. Rest becomes deeper.

DECEMBER 5

Rest Without Guilt

Rest can feel undeserved when productivity has been prioritized for long periods. Today invites you to rest without needing to justify it. Permission restores balance.

Resting without guilt does not mean neglecting responsibility. It means recognizing rest as necessary rather than optional. This recognition supports renewal.

As you move through the day, notice moments when guilt arises around rest. Allow yourself to rest anyway. Renewal strengthens through acceptance.

Guilt-free rest restores energy. It calms the nervous system. Renewal becomes sustainable.

DECEMBER 6

Honor End-Year Fatigue

Fatigue often accumulates quietly over months of effort and responsibility. Today invites you to acknowledge tiredness without judgment or resistance. Recognition supports rest.

Honoring end-year fatigue does not mean giving up or disengaging. It means allowing your body and mind to signal the need for care. This acknowledgment restores balance.

As you move through the day, notice where fatigue is present. Allow yourself to respond with gentleness rather than pressure. Renewal grows through respect.

Fatigue honored becomes informative. It guides restoration. Rest deepens naturally.

DECEMBER 7

Practice Deep Rest

Deep rest goes beyond physical stillness and reaches mental and emotional layers. Today invites you to allow rest that is uninterrupted and unproductive. Depth restores renewal.

Practicing deep rest does not require sleep or isolation. It means allowing moments where nothing is demanded of you. This openness supports healing.

As you move through the day, notice opportunities for deeper rest. Allow yourself to enter them fully. Renewal grows through stillness.

Deep rest replenishes reserves. It quiets inner noise. Renewal feels tangible.

DECEMBER 8

Reflect on Wins

Wins are often overlooked when attention remains on what remains unfinished. Today invites you to reflect on accomplishments both large and small. Recognition restores confidence.

Reflecting on wins does not require comparison or justification. It means acknowledging effort, growth, and perseverance. This acknowledgment supports renewal.

As you move through the day, notice moments where progress becomes visible. Allow yourself to recognize those wins. Renewal grows through affirmation.

Acknowledged wins reinforce resilience. They restore motivation. Renewal feels deserved.

DECEMBER 9

Close Emotional Loops

Unresolved emotions can linger quietly and drain energy. Today invites you to notice where emotional closure is possible. Awareness supports rest.

Closing emotional loops does not require confrontation or explanation. It means allowing feelings to complete their course internally. This completion restores calm.

As you move through the day, notice emotions that feel unfinished. Allow yourself to process them gently. Renewal grows through resolution.

Emotional closure frees energy. It reduces weight. Rest becomes more complete.

DECEMBER 10

Welcome Quiet Moments

Quiet moments often appear briefly and pass unnoticed. Today invites you to welcome stillness when it arises. Quiet supports renewal.

Welcoming quiet moments does not require silence or isolation. It means allowing calm to be felt when it appears. This allowance restores balance.

As you move through the day, notice moments of quiet between activity. Allow yourself to rest there briefly. Renewal grows through presence.

Quiet moments settle the nervous system. They restore clarity. Renewal deepens gently.

DECEMBER 11

Restore Inner Peace

Inner peace often returns when external demands soften. Today invites you to notice where calm is already present beneath surface activity. Awareness restores steadiness.

Restoring inner peace does not require eliminating all challenges. It means allowing yourself to feel settled even when life remains imperfect. This allowance supports renewal.

As you move through the day, notice moments when your inner state feels calm. Allow yourself to rest there briefly. Renewal grows through recognition.

Inner peace stabilizes emotion. It reduces reactivity. Renewal feels grounding.

DECEMBER 12

Prepare for Renewal

Preparation for renewal begins with awareness rather than action. Today invites you to notice what feels ready to shift or begin anew. Reflection supports readiness.

Preparing for renewal does not require plans or resolutions. It means creating internal space for what comes next. This openness supports balance.

As you move through the day, notice thoughts or feelings about new beginnings. Allow yourself to acknowledge them gently. Renewal grows through preparation.

Preparation softens transition. It reduces uncertainty. Renewal feels supported.

DECEMBER 13

Let the Year Settle

The year holds many experiences that need time to settle fully. Today invites you to allow memories and lessons to rest without analysis. Settling supports closure.

Letting the year settle does not require reviewing every detail. It means allowing what has happened to be complete. This completion supports rest.

As you move through the day, notice when reflection feels quiet rather than active. Allow yourself to remain there. Renewal grows through stillness.

Settled experience becomes wisdom. It reduces mental noise. Rest deepens naturally.

DECEMBER 14

Breathe in Closure

Closure often arrives through small moments of acknowledgment. Today invites you to use breath as a way to recognize endings gently. Breathing supports calm.

Breathing in closure does not require finality or certainty. It means allowing yourself to feel the completion of a chapter. This feeling supports renewal.

As you move through the day, notice moments when something feels finished. Allow yourself to breathe into that awareness. Renewal grows through acceptance.

Closure through breath softens emotion. It releases tension. Rest becomes accessible.

DECEMBER 15

Reflect Without Regret

Reflection feels lighter when regret is released. Today invites you to look back with understanding rather than self-criticism. Compassion supports renewal.

Reflecting without regret does not mean denying mistakes or pain. It means allowing learning to exist without blame. This approach restores balance.

As you move through the day, notice memories that carry emotional weight. Allow yourself to meet them with kindness. Renewal grows through compassion.

Compassionate reflection heals. It restores clarity. Renewal feels gentle.

DECEMBER 16

Choose Gentle Endings

Endings feel more supportive when approached with care rather than urgency. Today invites you to notice where softness can replace pressure as things conclude. Gentleness restores calm.

Choosing gentle endings does not require avoiding completion. It means allowing closure to arrive without force. This approach supports rest.

As you move through the day, notice moments that feel ready to end. Allow yourself to let them close kindly. Renewal grows through gentleness.

Gentle endings reduce tension. They honor experience. Rest becomes deeper.

DECEMBER 17

Release Lingering Tension

Tension can remain in the body and mind even when activity slows. Today invites you to notice where holding on is unnecessary. Awareness restores ease.

Releasing lingering tension does not require specific techniques or effort. It means allowing relaxation to happen naturally. This allowance supports renewal.

As you move through the day, notice areas of tightness or strain. Allow yourself to soften them gently. Renewal grows through release.

Released tension frees energy. It restores comfort. Rest feels more complete.

DECEMBER 18

Appreciate How Far You've Come

Progress often becomes clearer when you pause to look back. Today invites you to appreciate growth without comparison or judgment. Recognition restores confidence.

Appreciating how far you have come does not require measuring success. It means acknowledging persistence, effort, and change. This acknowledgment supports renewal.

As you move through the day, notice moments that reflect progress. Allow yourself to recognize them fully. Renewal grows through appreciation.

Recognized progress strengthens resilience. It affirms worth. Renewal feels earned.

DECEMBER 19

Allow Deep Stillness

Stillness offers restoration when it is allowed rather than forced. Today invites you to notice moments when quiet naturally arises. Allowing supports rest.

Allowing deep stillness does not require isolation or silence. It means letting the mind and body settle together. This settling supports renewal.

As you move through the day, notice moments when stillness feels accessible. Allow yourself to remain there. Renewal grows through stillness.

Deep stillness calms the nervous system. It restores clarity. Rest becomes profound.

DECEMBER 20

Simplify Final Days

Simplicity supports ease as the year draws toward its close. Today invites you to notice where simplifying reduces strain. Awareness restores balance.

Simplifying final days does not require removing everything. It means choosing what truly matters and letting the rest go. This discernment supports rest.

As you move through the day, notice opportunities to simplify. Allow yourself to choose ease over excess. Renewal grows through simplicity.

Simplified days feel lighter. They preserve energy. Rest becomes sustainable.

DECEMBER 21

Rest Body and Mind

Rest becomes more complete when both body and mind are allowed to slow together. Today invites you to notice where mental activity continues even when physical rest begins. Awareness restores balance.

Resting body and mind does not require complete stillness or silence. It means allowing thoughts to soften alongside physical relaxation. This coordination supports renewal.

As you move through the day, notice moments when both body and mind feel calmer. Allow yourself to remain there briefly. Renewal grows through alignment.

Balanced rest restores energy. It reduces fatigue. Renewal feels integrated.

DECEMBER 22

Sit With Gratitude

Gratitude can be felt quietly without needing expression or action. Today invites you to sit with appreciation as a steady presence. Stillness supports awareness.

Sitting with gratitude does not require listing or reflection. It means allowing thankfulness to be felt in the body and mind. This presence supports renewal.

As you move through the day, notice moments when gratitude arises naturally. Allow yourself to stay with it gently. Renewal grows through feeling.

Felt gratitude calms the nervous system. It stabilizes emotion. Renewal feels grounded.

DECEMBER 23

Welcome Calm

Calm often appears subtly rather than dramatically. Today invites you to notice where calm is already present beneath activity. Awareness restores ease.

Welcoming calm does not require removing all stimulation. It means allowing steadiness to be noticed and valued. This welcome supports renewal.

As you move through the day, notice moments when calm surfaces briefly. Allow yourself to receive it fully. Renewal grows through acceptance.

Calm settles the mind. It reduces reactivity. Renewal feels accessible.

DECEMBER 24

Let Go Fully

Letting go can feel more complete when it is intentional. Today invites you to notice where holding on no longer serves you. Awareness restores lightness.

Letting go fully does not require understanding or explanation. It means releasing without revisiting or reclaiming. This release supports rest.

As you move through the day, notice what feels ready to be released entirely. Allow yourself to let it go gently. Renewal grows through completion.

Full release restores clarity. It reduces inner weight. Rest becomes deeper.

DECEMBER 25

Create Year-End Ritual

Ritual provides structure for reflection and closure. Today invites you to create a simple practice that honors the end of the year. Intention supports renewal.

Creating a year-end ritual does not require formality or tradition. It means choosing an action that feels meaningful to you. This choice supports completion.

As you move through the day, notice what kind of ritual feels supportive. Allow yourself to engage with care. Renewal grows through intention.

Ritual anchors reflection. It marks transition. Renewal feels held.

DECEMBER 26

Reflect With Compassion

Reflection becomes healing when compassion leads the process. Today invites you to look back on experiences with understanding rather than judgment. Kindness restores balance.

Reflecting with compassion does not mean avoiding truth or difficulty. It means allowing empathy for yourself alongside honesty. This balance supports renewal.

As you move through the day, notice memories that arise during reflection. Allow yourself to meet them gently. Renewal grows through kindness.

Compassionate reflection softens regret. It restores clarity. Renewal feels supportive.

DECEMBER 27

Honor Your Effort

Effort deserves acknowledgment, especially when it has gone unseen. Today invites you to recognize the energy you have given throughout the year. Recognition restores worth.

Honoring your effort does not require comparison or external validation. It means acknowledging perseverance and commitment internally. This acknowledgment supports renewal.

As you move through the day, notice moments when effort becomes visible in hindsight. Allow yourself to honor it fully. Renewal grows through recognition.

Honored effort builds confidence. It affirms resilience. Renewal feels deserved.

DECEMBER 28

Choose Rest Over Rush

The impulse to rush can return even during times meant for rest. Today invites you to choose rest intentionally when urgency appears. Choice restores calm.

Choosing rest over rush does not mean ignoring responsibility. It means prioritizing steadiness over speed. This choice supports renewal.

As you move through the day, notice moments when rushing feels unnecessary. Allow yourself to slow deliberately. Renewal grows through intention.

Restful choice calms the nervous system. It reduces pressure. Renewal feels sustainable.

DECEMBER 29

End With Kindness

Kindness can shape how experiences are remembered and integrated. Today invites you to approach endings with gentleness toward yourself and others. Gentleness supports renewal.

Ending with kindness does not require resolution or agreement. It means allowing compassion to guide closure. This approach preserves calm.

As you move through the day, notice moments when kindness influences how things conclude. Allow yourself to act with care. Renewal grows through gentleness.

Kind endings soften memory. They reduce emotional residue. Renewal feels peaceful.

DECEMBER 30

Welcome Renewal

Renewal begins quietly as space opens after rest and reflection. Today invites you to notice where readiness for something new is emerging. Awareness supports transition.

Welcoming renewal does not require action or commitment. It means allowing openness to form naturally. This openness supports balance.

As you move through the day, notice feelings of readiness or curiosity about what comes next. Allow yourself to acknowledge them gently. Renewal grows through openness.

Renewal feels subtle at first. It brings quiet energy. Transition becomes natural.